Walther's
ORTHODONTIC Notes

Walther's Orthodontic Notes

W. J. B. HOUSTON
FDS RCS (Edin) PhD, DOrth

*Professor of Orthodontics,
United Medical and Dental Schools
of Guy's and St. Thomas's Hospitals
(University of London)*

Fourth Edition

WRIGHT

London Boston Singapore Sydney Toronto Wellington

Wright
is an imprint of Butterworth Scientific

All rights reserved. No part of this publication may be reproduced in any material form (including photocopying or storing it in any medium by electronic means and whether or not transiently or incidentally to some other use of this publication) without the written permission of the copyright owner except in accordance with the provisions of the Copyright, Designs and Patents Act 1988 or under the terms of a licence issued by the Copyright Licensing Agency Ltd, 33–34 Alfred Place, London, England WC1E 7DP. Applications for the copyright owner's written permission to reproduce any part of this publication should be addressed to the Publishers.

Warning: The doing of an unauthorised act in relation to a copyright work may result in both a civil claim for damages and criminal prosecution.

This book is sold subject to the Standard Conditions of Sale of Net Books and may not be re-sold in the UK below the net price given by the Publishers in their current price list.

© **Butterworth & Co. (Publishers) Ltd, 1990**

First edition, 1960
Reprinted, 1962
Reprinted, 1965
Second edition, 1967
Reprinted, 1972
Third edition, 1976
Reprinted, 1979
Fourth edition, 1983
Reprinted, 1985
Reprinted, 1990

British Library Cataloguing in Publication Data
Walther, D. P.
  Walther's orthodontic notes.—4th ed.
  1. Orthodontic
  I. Title   II. Houston, W. J. B.
  617.6'43   RK521

ISBN 0 7236 0670 6

Library of Congress Catalog Card Number: 82-62623

Printed and bound by Hartnolls Ltd, Bodmin, Cornwall

Preface to the Fourth Edition

Since its first appearance in 1960, *Orthodontic Notes* has become a popular text with undergraduates. Although it has been reviewed extensively since that time, the intentions of Professor Walther have been followed: to present in a clear and concise fashion, the essentials of orthodontics required by undergraduate dental students and general dental practitioners. The brevity of presentation precludes detailed discussion of the many controversial topics in orthodontics. However, such debates are liable to be confusing rather than informative for the student who is being introduced to a subject. Thus a particular viewpoint is presented—hopefully a consistent and commonsense framework of ideas. This should provide an adequate theoretical basis for the undergraduate student or general dental practitioner, and should form a sound foundation for the student who wishes to go further and to specialize in orthodontics.

W. J. B. H.

From the Preface to the First Edition

These orthodontic notes are taken from the lectures given to the students at the Royal Dental Hospital, School of Dental Surgery, London. They are published in the hope that they may be of use to others as well.

They are intended to form a basis around which both the undergraduate and postgraduate can read and develop this subject. Nothing original is claimed in these notes, in which I have tried to put forward up-to-date views and their application to modern orthodontics.

Numerous textbooks, articles and papers published on the subject have all been immensely useful, and I would like to express my thanks to their various authors and contributors. I would especially like to express my grateful thanks to the various members of the staff of the Royal and the other London dental hospitals and schools of which I have been a member, namely the Eastman Dental Hospital, Guy's Hospital, and the Hospital for Sick Children, Great Ormond Street.

D. P. W.

Contributors

D. A. Plint BDS D ORTH FDS RCS
Consultant Orthodontist
The Hospital for Sick Children
Great Ormond Street
London

Clefts of the Lip and Palate—Chapter 20

M. J. C. Wake MB CHB FDS RCS BDS
Consultant Oral Surgeon
The Queen Elizabeth Hospital
The Queen Elizabeth Medical Centre
Edgbaston
Birmingham

Oral Surgery in Relation to Orthodontics—Chapter 19

Contents

1	Introduction	1
2	The Facial Skeleton	5
3	Soft Tissue Morphology and Behaviour	27
4	Mandibular Positions and Paths of Closure	34
5	Development of Normal Occlusion	36
6	Malocclusion	46
7	Tissue Changes with Tooth Movement	54
8	Principles and Components of Removable Appliances	61
9	Removable Appliances	74
10	Local Factors in the Aetiology of Malocclusion	94
11	Tooth-Arch Disproportion	118
12	Arch Malrelationship	128
13	Class I Malocclusions	135
14	Class II Division 1 Malocclusions	138
15	Class II Division 2 Malocclusions	147
16	Class III Malocclusions	154
17	Fixed Appliances	163
18	Functional Appliances	172
19	Oral Surgery in Relation to Orthodontics	177
20	Clefts of the Lip and Palate	190
	Appendix I: Orthodontic Diagnosis and Treatment Planning	201
	Appendix II: Definitions	204
	Index	209

Chapter 1

Introduction

Although the terminology in this text has been kept as simple as possible, it is necessary at the outset to define a few fundamental concepts.

Orthodontics is that branch of dental science concerned with genetic variations, development and growth of facial forms and the manner in which these factors affect the occlusion of the teeth and the function of associated organs. Thus while orthodontic techniques are concerned with the treatment of irregularities of the teeth, the study of orthodontics includes the growth, development and function of the whole orofacial complex.

Ideal occlusion is a hypothetical concept based on the anatomy of the teeth. It is rarely if ever found in nature. However, it provides a standard by which other occlusions can be judged.

Normal occlusion (*Fig.* 1.1) is commonly described as 'An occlusion within the accepted deviation of the ideal'. This vague definition means that there are no clear limits to the range of normal occlusion. In general, minor variations in the alignment of the teeth which are not of aesthetic or functional importance are consistent with a normal occlusion.

Malocclusion is an irregularity in the occlusion beyond the accepted range of normal. The fact that an individual has a malocclusion is not in itself a justification for treatment. Only if it is possible to say with certainty that the patient will benefit, aesthetically or functionally, and only if he is suitable and willing to undergo treatment, should orthodontic intervention be considered.

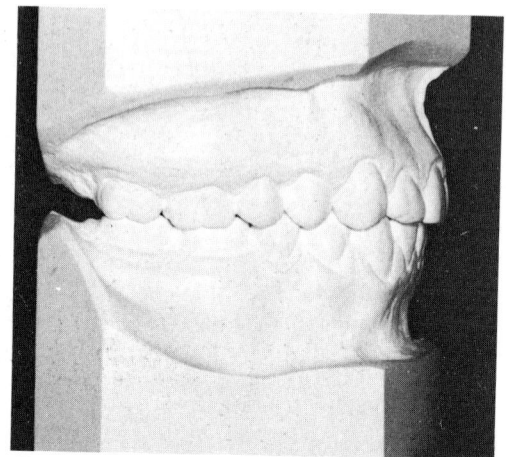

Fig. 1.1. Normal occlusion of the permanent teeth.

The Scope and Aims of Orthodontic Treatment

1. The improvement of facial and dental aesthetics.
2. The alignment of the teeth to eliminate stagnation areas.
3. The elimination of premature contacts which give rise to mandibular displacements and may cause later muscle or joint pain.
4. The elimination of traumatic irregularities of the teeth (*Fig.* 1.2).
5. The alignment of prominent teeth which are liable to be damaged.
6. The alignment of irregular teeth prior to bridge-work, crowns or partial dentures.

The Timing of Orthodontic Treatment

The Deciduous Dentition

Treatment at this stage is hardly ever indicated. The only possible exception is where a malpositioned tooth gives rise to marked mandibular displacement.

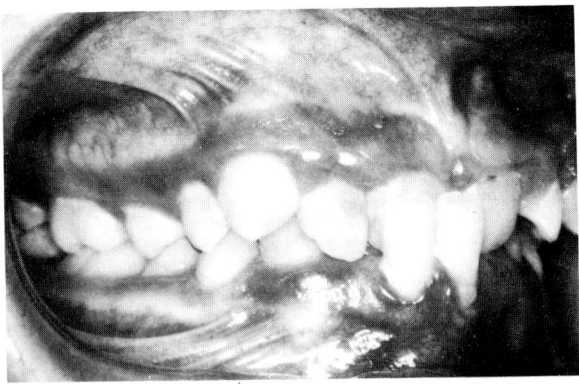

Fig. 1.2. A traumatic occlusion. Note the gingival recession on the lower central incisors.

The Early Mixed Dentition

The planned extraction of extensively carious first permanent molars (p. 105), balancing extractions of deciduous teeth (p. 99) and serial extractions are undertaken during this stage. Space maintainers (p. 99) may be fitted and simple orthodontic treatment to correct an instanding incisor or eliminate a mandibular displacement (p. 133) may be indicated. Only treatment which can be completed rapidly and which will be stable should be begun. Prolonged appliance wear is to be avoided.

The Late Mixed and Early Permanent Dentition

At this stage, the greater part of orthodontic treatment is carried out: most of the permanent teeth have erupted; there is little further growth in arch width and so crowding can reliably be estimated; in the majority of children the jaw relationship changes only to a small extent after the age of 10 years (Chapter 2) and so it is possible to plan and carry out orthodontic treatment in confidence that major growth changes are not likely to affect treatment adversely. Furthermore, children in this age group are often more willing to wear appliances than are adults.

The Late Permanent Dentition

Although orthodontic treatment can be undertaken at any age adults are often unwilling to wear appliances over a prolonged period. It is usually wise to limit treatment to simple procedures which can be completed in a short time span.

Chapter 2

The Facial Skeleton

GROWTH OF THE FACE AND SKULL

The bones of the cranial vault develop in the membranes covering the brain in the embryo. Centres of ossification appear and the bones expand so that by birth they are related to one another at sutures although some areas, the fontanelles, still have a membranous covering (*Fig.* 2.1). The sutures are sites at which limited movement of the bones is possible and where growth in the size of the cranial vault can occur. They are fibrous joints with little inherent growth potential: growth at the sutures occurs by their expansion due to growth in volume of the cranial contents. In addition to the increase in surface area, the bones of the cranial vault are thickened as a result of periosteal apposition. They consist of outer and inner tables of compact bone separated by a layer of cancellous bone. Where functional demands require, for example at muscle attachments and sites of stress concentration, the outer table may be elevated into ridges and crests. This happens at the temporal and nuchal crests and at the supra-orbital ridges where the space between the inner and outer tables becomes pneumatized.

The cranial base comprises the bones that develop from the cartilaginous chondrocranium of the embryo. At birth, cartilage remains at sites where growth can occur: the synchondroses whose structure resembles that of the epiphyseal cartilages of the long bones, except that growth occurs in both the bones contributing to the joint. The spheno-ethmoidal and spheno-occipital synchondroses are responsible for growth in length of the cranial base.

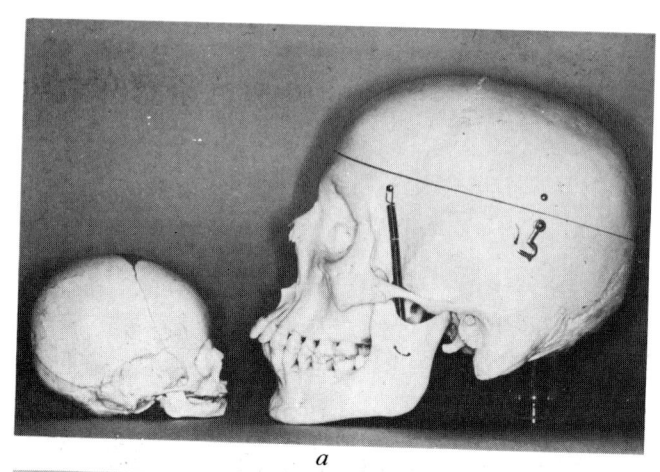

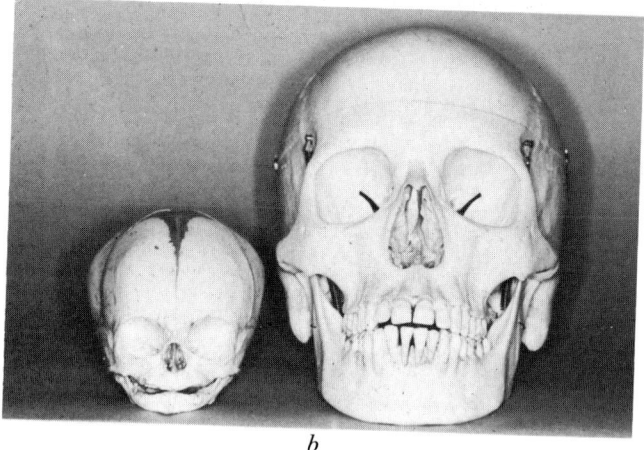

Fig. 2.1. Neonate and adult skulls. Note the differences in proportions between facial skeleton and calvarium at the different ages. The proportions of the facial skeleton also change with age.

The former fuses at about six years of age after which there is little growth change at the midline in the floor of the anterior cranial fossa. This relatively stable area of the anterior cranial base is used as a reference structure from

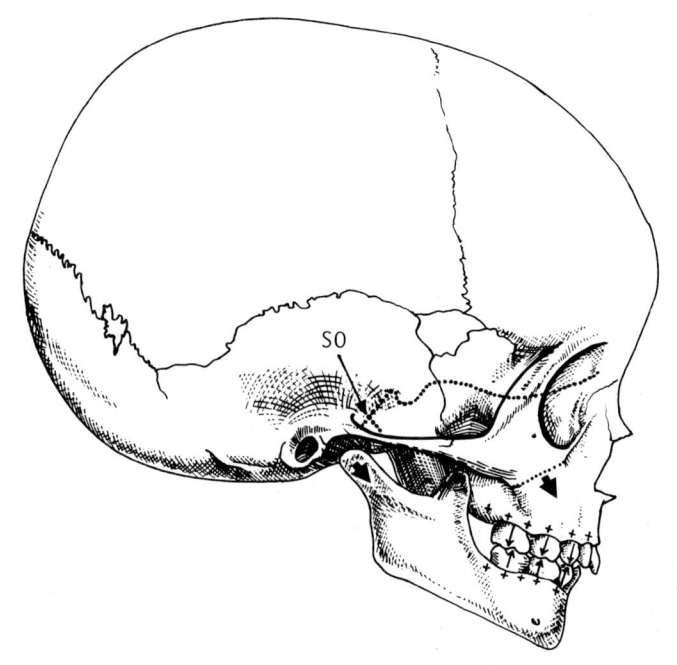

Fig. 2.2. The maxilla grows downwards and forwards in part due to growth at sutures (i.e. displacement) and in part by surface apposition and remodelling of bone (i.e. drift). The mandible grows downwards and forwards from its cranial articulations at a greater rate than does the maxilla. Thus the intermaxillary space grows in height and is bridged by vertical growth at the alveolar processes and eruption of the teeth. The midline cranial base is indicated by a dotted line. Growth at the spheno-occipital synchondrosis (SO) increases the distance between the cranial articulations of the maxilla and mandible.

which growth changes elsewhere in the facial skeleton can be measured. The upper facial skeleton is related to the anterior cranial fossa while the mandible is related to the middle cranial fossa at its articulation with the temporal bone (*Fig.* 2.2). The length of the cranial base thus has an influence on jaw relationships, and growth at the spheno-occipital synchondrosis, which continues until about the age of puberty, has an influence on jaw relationships. Growth of the cranial base is not influenced by orthodontic means and is probably under fairly tight genetic control.

The Facial Skeleton

The maxilla grows downwards and forwards from the anterior cranial base, in part as a result of growth at the circum-maxillary suture system and in part as a result of extensive surface apposition and remodelling of bone. In general terms the outward and downward facing surfaces of the maxilla are formative, in particular at the alveolar process and on the oral surface of the palate, with corresponding resorption on the nasal surfaces. Thus the maxilla grows downwards and forwards in part due to drift (surface remodelling). The sutures of the upper facial skeleton are structurally comparable with those of the cranial vault and, like them, probably have little independent growth potential. However, it has not been possible to isolate the primary growth-promoting forces in the upper facial skeleton. Growth of the nasal septum and the eyeballs have been cited as possible factors. Probably no single factor controls and directs growth of the upper facial skeleton. It has been shown that heavy forces applied to the maxillary teeth by orthodontic appliances can, according to the direction of traction, reduce or accelerate growth at the maxillary sutures. However, this is of limited practical application because, following such treatment, the natural growth pattern tends to reassert itself and there is a corresponding catch-up or lag so that the ultimate facial pattern is little affected. Only if such treatment were continued for many years until facial growth was nearly complete would lasting appreciable changes be achieved.

Growth in the overall length of the mandible takes place largely at the condyle, but of course comparable remodelling periosteal growth changes take place to maintain the form of the mandible. It is a question of continuing controversy whether growth at the condyles propels the mandible downwards and forwards from the glenoid fossa or whether condylar growth is merely adaptive to other factors that carry the mandible downwards and forwards. It seems probable that the condylar cartilage has an appreciable inherent growth potential but that it can be affected by local factors. However, its growth can be influenced only to a very limited extent by orthodontic appliance treatment. Proponents of functional appliances (Chapter 18) claim that condylar growth can be controlled but this is still a matter of debate. The general practitioner is wise to plan treatment on the assumption that his appliances will not influence condylar growth.

The mandible grows downwards and forwards from its articulation with the middle cranial fossa, faster than does the maxilla (*Fig.* 2.2). Antero-posteriorly this is largely compensated for by the growth of the spheno-occipital synchondrosis which carries the maxilla forward. However, the tendency is for mandibular prognathism (i.e. projection from under the cranial structures) to increase slightly faster than does maxillary prognathism. Vertically the distance between the mandibular and maxillary bases, the intermaxillary space, increases in height. This is bridged by vertical growth of the teeth and alveolar processes which adapt to changes in height and shape of the intermaxillary space.

The vertical relationship of the mandible to the upper facial structures is determined not only by growth at the condyles, but by the lengths of the muscles and fascia attached to it: principally the muscles of mastication passing between the mandible and the rest of the craniofacial skeleton and the suprahyoid muscles below. Growth in length of these is in turn influenced by growth in length of the neck and the cervical vertebrae. Many other factors, such as the physiological need to maintain an airway, play a part in determining mandibular positions. This means

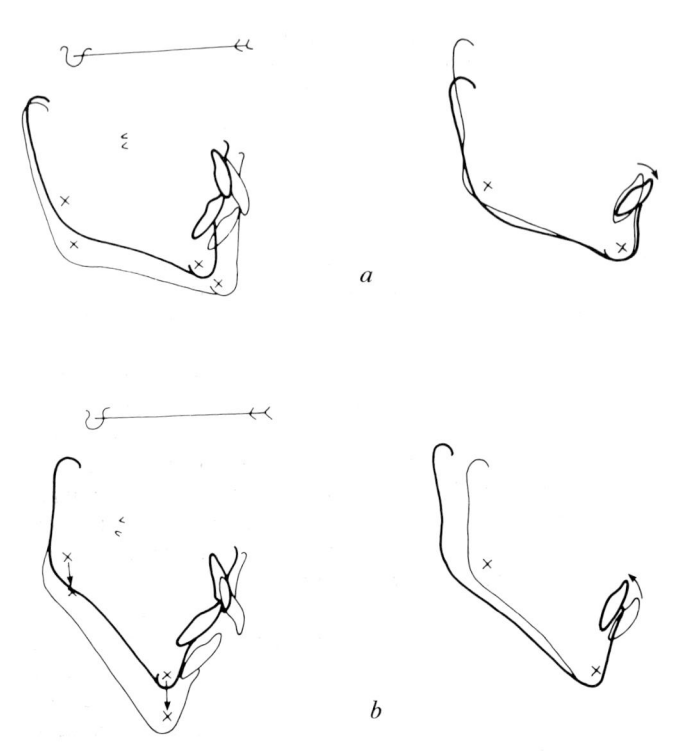

Fig. 2.3. Mandibular growth rotations: *a*, anterior growth rotation; *b*, posterior growth rotation. The crosses indicate hypothetical stable points in the mandible, purely for the purposes of illustration. Where the posterior and anterior facial heights grow to different extents a mandibular growth rotation will occur but will to a large extent be masked by remodelling at the lower and posterior borders of the mandible. This is revealed when mandibular outlines are superimposed on the stable structures. The relative orientation of the lower incisors within the face is maintained to a large extent by dento-alveolar adaptation. In most children, growth rotations are small.

that superimposed on the downward and forward translation of the mandible relative to the cranial base, there may be minor degrees of anterior or posterior rotation (*Fig.* 2.3) depending on the balance of growth between the condyle and the muscles attached to the mandible. As discussed below, the position of the teeth and alveolar structures adapts to these changes in mandibular relationships.

Patterns of Growth

At birth, the volume of the brain case is greater than that of the face (*Fig.* 2.1) but after the age of 6 years, there is little further growth in volume because the brain has nearly reached its adult size. The facial skeleton grows steadily over a much longer period and thus in the adult forms a much larger proportion of the skull than in the child and projects further forward from under the brain case (*Fig.* 2.1). The infant's face is relatively broad but with postnatal growth, the proportions of the face change, growth in breadth being least, and in depth most. Thus on average the face in an adult appears longer and narrower and projects further forward than in the child. Some of the most noticeable changes in facial characteristics are due to the fact that the eyes are relatively large in the infant but, like the brain, grow relatively little after the age of 6 years while the nose is very much more prominent in the adult than in the child. These changes do not affect the occlusion but changes in the character of the face obviously affect the appearance of the dentition in the face: even with a normal occlusion, the teeth of the 9-year-old child may seem to be rather large and prominent but with growth of the rest of the face and in particular of the nose, the impression changes.

Facial Growth and the Occlusion

The alveolar bone is highly adaptable, depending for its presence and location on the presence and position of the teeth: remove a tooth and the associated alveolar process resorbs; move a tooth and it remodels.

Dento-alveolar Compensation

Because the upper and lower teeth erupt into the common zone between lips, cheeks and tongue they tend to be guided towards one another to establish an occlusion and to compensate for any transverse or antero-posterior malrelationships of the jaws. Variations in vertical jaw relationships are compensated by a greater or lesser degree or eruption of the teeth and growth of the alveolar processes. Where the skeletal malrelationships are too severe, the dento-alveolar compensation described above may not be sufficient to establish a normal occlusion and so crossbite, open bite and antero-posterior arch malrelationships may develop. However, arch malrelationships will often be less severe than might have been expected from the jaw malrelationship (see Fig. 2.4c). In some cases dento-alveolar compensation does not operate because of variations in soft tissue patterns. For example, if the upper lip is short and the lips are habitually parted the upper incisors will tend to be proclined and are not guided towards the lower incisors. The lower incisors will then continue to erupt, possibly until they contact the palate. Dento-alveolar compensation is not always advantageous: in some cases of mandibular retrusion for example, compensation occurs by retroclination of the upper incisors

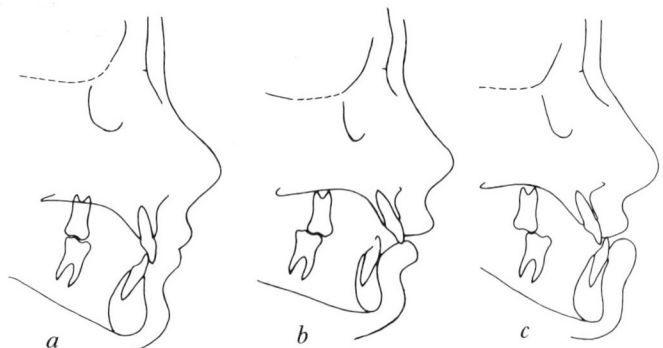

Fig. 2.4. Skeletal patterns: *a,* Class I; *b,* Class II; *c, Class III.*

(*see Fig.* 15.1). This type of incisor relationship is usually associated with a deep overbite and may be traumatic as well as being unsightly.

Dento-alveolar Adaptation

As the face grows, the intermaxillary space increases in height and antero-posterior jaw relationships may change. As a result of vertical growth of the teeth and alveolar processes, occlusal contacts and the soft tissue environment of the teeth, the existing occlusion or malocclusion tends to be maintained. Dento-alveolar adaptation is a dynamic process while dento-alveolar compensation refers to an existing state of affairs: on examining a patient, it is possible to ascertain to what extent dento-alveolar compensation exists. Only with records obtained on more than one occasion can one identify the nature and amount of dento-alveolar adaptation that may have occurred over that time period.

Dento-alveolar adaptation is greatest vertically, in response to vertical growth of the intermaxillary space. Little change in transverse jaw relationships occurs with growth. Where changes in antero-posterior jaw relationships occur there will usually be corresponding dento-alveolar adaptation. Most commonly the mandible grows forwards slightly more than the maxilla and the upper incisors procline while the lower incisors retrocline. The proclination of the upper incisors does not produce spacing because the upper buccal segments come forward by a comparable amount. Retroclination of the lower incisors usually results in crowding. If the adaptive mechanisms cannot cope with the extent of the change in jaw relationships there will be occlusal change. This most often happens where there is a Class III arch relationship (*see Fig.* 2.4*c*) and there is little or no incisor overbite.

Growth rotations of the mandible may be superimposed upon the changes described above. Such growth rotations initiate dento-alveolar adaptation which may in turn lead to lower incisor crowding. With a posterior growth rotation (*Fig.* 2.3*b*) the lower incisors tend to become retroclined under the influence of the soft tissue integument of the face so that their relationship to upper facial reference planes changes little. The buccal segments do not move back by a corresponding amount and so lower arch crowding may appear or become more severe.

Anterior mandibular growth rotations (*Fig.* 2.3*a*) are associated with proclination of the lower incisors within the alveolar process and with an upward and forward path of eruption of the buccal teeth. Measured to a reference plane in the upper face, the lower incisors do not become proclined but maintain their inclination. Provided that the forward movement of anterior and posterior teeth are in balance there should be no change in the space conditions of the lower arch. However, the lower incisors, through contact with the upper incisors, are often prevented from adapting completely, particularly if at the same time the mandible is growing forwards to a greater extent than is the maxilla. In these circumstances the lower buccal teeth will encroach on space for the lower labial segment with the development of lower incisor crowding.

Orthodontic treatment planning for the child is based on the hypothesis that the growth changes which take place will be within the normal range and so will have only minor effects on the occlusion. This is satisfactory for the majority of patients but occasionally unforeseen changes may occur and treatment planning will have to be revised. Many attempts have been made to predict accurately the future growth trends of the facial skeleton in the individual, but at the present time this is not possible.

SKELETAL RELATIONSHIP

The relationship between the jaws has important effects on dental arch relationship. Unless lateral skull radiographs are available (*see Fig.* 2.6), jaw relationship is assessed from the clinical examination of the patient. Skeletal relationships should be considered in three axes: antero-posterior, vertical and transverse.

Clinical Assessment
Antero-posterior

This sagittal relationship between the jaws (the skeletal pattern) depends on the length of maxilla, length of mandible and the length of the cranial base between its articulation with the maxilla and the temporomandibular joint. The skeletal pattern is assessed by examining the profile as the patient sits unsupported, with the head in the free postural position and the mandible in the rest position or with the teeth in centric occlusion (the mandible must not be postured or displaced). When the mandible is normally related to the maxilla the skeletal pattern is Class I; when it is posteriorly positioned relative to the maxilla the skeletal pattern is Class II; and when it is too far forward the skeletal pattern is Class III (*Fig.* 2.4). Subjective assessment of this sort is open to error and if there is a marked discrepancy between the thickness of the upper and lower lips, the soft tissue profile may give a misleading impression of the skeletal pattern. Nevertheless, this method of assessment is usually more accurate than attempts to judge skeletal relationships with the lips retracted. Minor variations in skeletal pattern are of little clinical importance and the larger variations from normal, which do have a bearing on aetiology and treatment, can readily be recognized.

Vertical

The space between the upper and lower skeletal bases is the intermaxillary space. The height of this space depends on the shape of the mandible and on the resting lengths of the muscles of mastication. Where the anterior height of

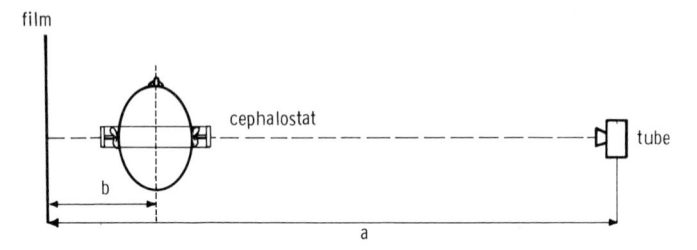

Fig. 2.5. When a cephalometric radiograph is obtained, the head is held in a fixed relationship to the film and X-ray tube. The ratio a/b determines the enlargement of the image.

the intermaxillary space is large an open bite may be found (Chapter 12).

The angle between Frankfort and mandibular planes (*Fig.* 2.7) gives an index of anterior intermaxillary height. The average value for this angle is 27° with a normal range of 5° in either direction. If the Frankfort mandibular planes angle is large the anterior intermaxillary height will usually be increased. It is not easy to estimate by eye the size of the Frankfort mandibular planes angle. Various forms of protractor are available but it is perhaps simpler to compare the lower and middle facial heights (*Fig.* 2.7). In the well-balanced face these heights should be equal. Clearly, the ratio between them will be affected by mid facial height but a relative increase in lower facial height may be associated with a skeletal open bite.

Transverse

The relative widths of the jaws have a bearing on the transverse relationship of the dental arches (Chapter 12). However, there is no way, clinically or radiologically, in which these widths can be measured. Discrepancies in skeletal base width usually have to be inferred from transverse malrelationships of the arches.

CEPHALOMETRIC ANALYSIS

Analysis of lateral skull radiographs allows a more detailed evaluation of facial structures than is possible from a visual assessment of facial appearance. The cephalometric lateral skull radiograph is taken with the head held in a specially designed holder (*Fig.* 2.5) so that there is a fixed constant relationship between the patient's head, the film and the anode of the X-ray tube: the midsagittal plane of the head should be parallel to and at a fixed distance from the film so that linear measurements are magnified by a known standard amount (usually about 10%). Some experience is required if a lateral skull radiograph is to be interpreted reliably. The features shown in *Fig.* 2.6 give a key to the general anatomy. Cephalometric landmarks can then be located (*Fig.* 2.7). The appearance of each landmark can vary appreciably between patients and some are much more difficult to identify reliably than are others. If the film is over-exposed it can be very difficult to locate the fine bony detail on the skeletal profile.

Definitions of Landmarks (Fig. 2.7)

Note: definitions using 'lowest' or 'highest' assume that the radiograph is orientated so that the Frankfort plane is horizontal.

Anterior nasal spine (ANS). The point of the bony nasal spine. The vertical level can be fixed quite reliably but the antero-posterior location may be difficult: the tip of the spine is thin and it may be overlaid by nasal cartilages which are nearly of the same radio-opacity.

Harvold recommended the use of points on the lower and upper contours of the spine where it was 3 mm thick. These may be more reliable than the traditional ANS but they may still be difficult to locate because the upper and lower margins of the spine are not always distinct.

Articulare (Ar). The point of intersection of the projection of the surface of the neck of the condyle and the inferior surface of the basi-occiput.

Basion (Ba). The most posterior inferior point in the

midline on the basi-occiput. This marks the posterior limit of the mid-line cranial base and lies on the anterior rim of foramen magnum.

Gonion (Go). The most posterior, inferior point on the angle of the mandible. It is located by drawing tangents to the angle of the mandible through menton and through articulare. Gonion lies where the bisector of the angle

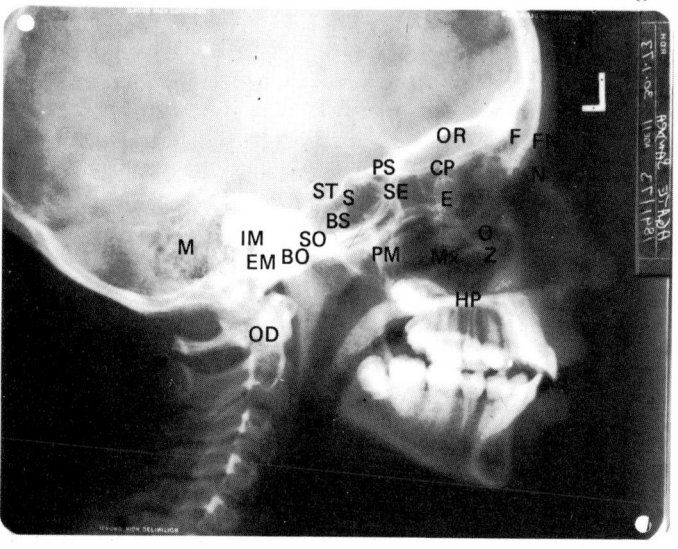

Fig. 2.6. A lateral skull radiograph illustrating the principal anatomical features.

BO = basi-occiput
BS = basi-phenoid
CP = cribriform plate of ethmoid
E = ethmoid air cells
EM = external acoustic meatus
F = frontal sinus
FN = fronto-nasal suture
HP = hard palate
IM = internal acoustic meatus
M = mastoid air cells
Mx = maxillary sinus
N = nasal bones

O = orbital margins
OD = odontoid process of axis
OR = orbital roof
PM = pterygomaxillary fissure
PS = planum sphenoidale
S = sphenoid air sinus
SE = site of spheno-ethmoidal synchondrosis
SO = spheno-occipital synchondrosis
ST = sella turcica, the pituitary fossa
Z = zygomatic process of maxilla

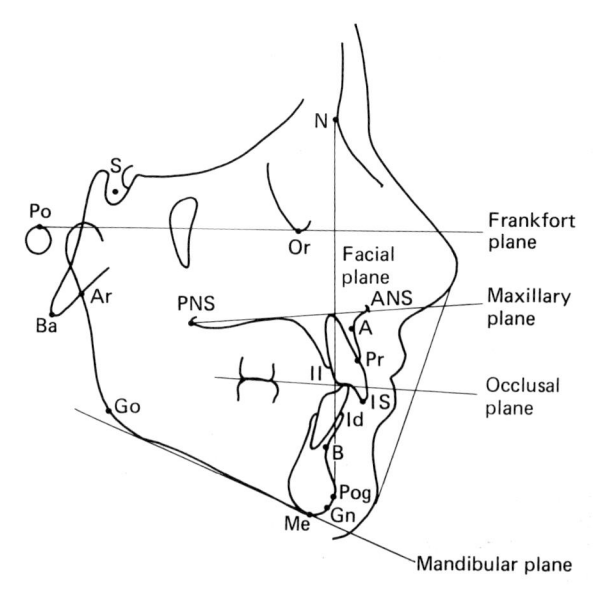

Fig. 2.7. Tracing of the radiograph shown in *Fig.* 2.6 indicating the main cephalometric landmarks (*see* text for definitions).

formed by these two tangents intersects the mandibular outline. This point may be used in drawing the mandibular plane and gonial angle. Where the outlines of the two sides do not coincide an 'average' outline should be drawn and the constructions related to this.

Gnathion (Gn). The most anterior, inferior point on the bony symphysis of the mandible. It is located where the bisector of the angle between the facial line (NPog) and the mandibular plane (through menton and tangent to the angle of the mandible) intersects the outline of the symphysis.

Incision inferius (II). The tip of the crown of the most prominent mandibular incisor.

Incision superius (IS). The tip of the crown of the most prominent maxillary incisor.

Infradentale (Id). The highest point on the alveolar crest labial to the most prominent lower incisor.

Menton (Me). The lowermost point on the mandibular symphysis.

Orbitale (Or). The most inferior point on the margin of the orbit. Strictly speaking, the left orbit should be used and some orthodontists use a radio-opaque pointer, or fix a marker to the skin before the radiograph is taken, to indicate this. When this is not done and two orbital borders are shown, the midpoint should be taken. Orbitale is difficult to locate with accuracy.

Posterior nasal spine (PNS). The tip of the posterior nasal spine can usually be seen unless unerupted molars obscure it. The outline of the palate gives a good indication of its vertical level and allows the maxillary plane to be drawn in. A line through the most inferior point on the pterygo-maxillary fissure, perpendicular to the maxillary plane, indicates the antero-posterior location of PNS.

Pogonion (Pog). The most anterior point of the bony chin.

Point A (A). Also known as subspinale, this is the deepest point on the maxillary profile between the anterior nasal spine and the alveolar crest. It can be difficult to locate if the maxillary profile is not clear: there may be a thin spine of bone extending downwards in the midline from the anterior nasal spine, or the shadow of the cheek can be superimposed. Point A is used to indicate the anterior limit of the maxillary base but it is not very reliable in this respect because the bone in this region remodels to some extent with orthodontic tooth movement, quite apart from the problems of locating the point. However, in spite of these difficulties, point A continues to be used because no entirely satisfactory alternative has been proposed.

Point B (B). Also known as supramentale, this is the mandibular point that corresponds to point A on the maxilla; however, it is more reliable. It is the deepest point on the concavity of the mandibular profile between the point of the chin and the alveolar crest. If the curvature is gentle, the vertical level of point B may be difficult to fix,

but this is not usually very important because it is used to measure antero-posterior jaw relationships.
Porion (Po). The highest point on the bony external acoustic meatus. If both sides are visible, the midpoint is taken. As already mentioned, porion can be very difficult to locate reliably. A useful guide is that the upper borders of the external acoustic meati should be on the same level as the articulating surfaces of the mandibular condyles, although these, too, are difficult to locate.
Prosthion (Pr). The lowest point on the alveolar crest labial to the most prominent upper central incisor.

Reference Lines and Planes (Fig. 2.7)

Cephalometric measurements will be described with the analyses, but certain widely used reference planes (or more correctly 'lines' as we are dealing with a two-dimensional representation) will be described here. A very large number of reference lines in the skull are described in the anthropological literature, but only a few of direct orthodontic importance will be mentioned.

Facial line (or plane). Nasion–pogonion. It indicates the general orientation of the facial profile.

Frankfort plane. Porion–orbitale. This plane is described as being horizontal when the head is in a free postural position. In fact, there is considerable individual variation. This, together with the unreliability of its end points and the fact that it represents no single coherent anatomical structure, means that there are serious reservations about its use as a reference structure.

Mandibular plane (Mn). A variety of lines has been used to indicate the orientation of the body of the mandible, but it probably makes little difference which is selected. The simplest to locate is the line from menton, tangent to the lower border of the mandible at the angle. The line Go–Gn is used by many but requires the construction of both points.

Maxillary plane (Mx). This line through the anterior and posterior nasal spines, indicates the orientation of the

palate. Where the anterior nasal spine curves upwards above the level of the nasal floor, it may be better to draw the maxillary plane through PNS parallel to the nasal floor.
Occlusal plane. Various definitions are offered. It may be represented by the line that passes through the occlusion of the mesial cusps of the most anterior permanent molars and halfway between the tips of the upper and lower central incisors. It is preferable to use a line following the occlusion of the molar and premolar teeth. This is known as the functional occlusal plane (FOP).

Many landmarks are a compromise between anatomical validity and the possibility of identification. For example, points A and B which are meant to represent maxillary and mandibular skeletal bases respectively are affected to a limited extent by tooth movement and alveolar remodelling. Thus cephalometric measurements must be interpreted with caution and too much emphasis should not be

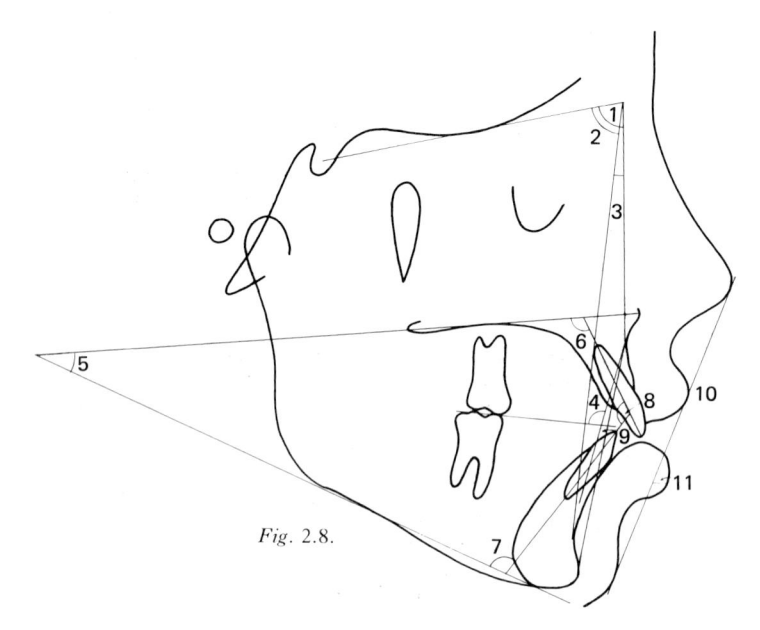

Fig. 2.8.

placed on minor variations in their values. If a cephalometric measurement is to have any meaning it is necessary to know the normal range of that measurement within the population group from which the patient comes (*see Fig. 2.8*). Even if one measurement is beyond the normal range it may be compensated for by other features and so it is necessary to look for a general pattern. The basic question is whether there is evidence of skeletal malrelationships and whether or not there has been dento-alveolar compensation. It is then possible to decide about the tooth movements that would be necessary to correct the arch malrelationships; and whether tipping movements (obtainable with a removable appliance) or controlled apical movement (requiring fixed appliances) will be appropriate. Where the skeletal discrepancy is severe, surgical

Fig. 2.8. Cephalometric analysis.

	Norms Mean ± Range		This case
1. SNA	82°	3	79
2. SNB	79°	3	72
3. ANB	3°	1	7
4. AB/FOP	90°	5	100
5. Max/Mand. Planes (MM)	27°	5	29
6. UI/Max. Plane	108°	5	110
7. LI/Mand. Plane	92°	5	102
8. UI/LI	133°	10	119
9. UI to A–Pog	0 mm	2	+4
10. Upper lip to Aesthetic Plane	0 mm		+1
11. Lower lip to Aesthetic Plane	0 mm		+4

Comments: Angle SNA is low but just within normal range while SNB is definitely low. Angle ANB at 7° indicates a definite Class II skeletal pattern and this is corroborated by the large angle between the line A–B and the Function Occlusal Plane. The upper incisors are at an average inclination to the maxillary plane while the lower incisors are proclined with the incisor edges in advance of the line A–Pog, indicating some dento-alveolar compensation for the Class II skeletal pattern. Vertically the jaw relationships are within normal limits. The lips were parted when the radiograph was taken, with the lower lip rather full and everted lying in advance of the Aesthetic Plane. It is important to assess clinically whether this correctly portrays the habitual lip posture.

correction may be considered. Treatment planning must never be undertaken using cephalometric analysis in isolation: the stability and aesthetic acceptability of the intended tooth movements can be fully evaluated only by reference to the soft tissue pattern and facial appearance of the living patient.

Measurement from Lateral Skull Radiographs

The relevant anatomical lines should be traced on to good quality tracing paper using a sharp, hard pencil. A very large number of cephalometric measurements has been proposed but, for the clinician, those shown in *Fig.* 2.8 give a comprehensive view of skeletal and dento-skeletal relationships.

The Interpretation of Cephalometric Measurements

Points A and B are taken to represent the anterior limits of the tooth-bearing areas of the maxilla and mandible. This relationship is usually assessed by reference to the anterior cranial base (S–N line). Angles SNA and SNB measure the prognathism, or projection in relation to the cranial base, of the maxilla and mandible. The difference between these (angle ANB) gives an indication of the jaw relationships as follows:

Angle ANB	*Skeletal class*
2–4 degrees	I
greater than 4 degrees	II
less than 2 degrees	III

This value can be misleading if the position of N is unusual but a warning of this may be given by a value of SNA that is unusually large or small. An alternative method of assessing the jaw relationship is to measure the angle between A and B and the functional occlusal plane (FOP). A problem with this measurement is that the orientation of the FOP varies greatly between individuals and can change with growth and treatment. However, it offers a useful check on the information given by angle ANB: if the two values are contradictory, then each should be interpreted with caution and a final judgement on skeletal relationships made from clinical observations.

As with direct clinical observation (*see* p. 16) the anterior height of the intermaxillary space may be estimated from the angle of the mandibular plane to the Frankfort plane, but as the latter is often difficult to locate on a radiograph the maxillary plane (ANS–PNS) is often used instead. On average, the Frankfort and maxillary planes are parallel to one another but they may diverge appreciably in some individuals.

Dento-skeletal Relationsnips

The inclinations of the upper incisors to the maxillary plane and of the lower incisors to the mandibular plane give an indication of whether or not any dento-alveolar compensation for anteroposterior skeletal discrepancies has taken place. They also give a guide to the type of tooth movements that will be required to correct incisor malrelationships. The distance of the most prominent lower incisor from the line between point A and the chin point (pogonion) is a guide to the position of the lower incisors relative to the lower skeletal profile. It is simpler to obtain a good incisor relationship and the appearance is usually better if the lower incisor edge lies close to the A–Pog line, than if it is far from it. However, this line should not be regarded as a treatment goal to the positioning of the lower incisors because it offers no guide to the position of stability.

The angle between the upper and lower incisors is related to the depth of overbite (except in Class III cases). A wide inter-incisor angle is usually associated with a deep overbite and if at the end of treatment this angle is too large, the overbite will usually deepen and may become traumatic (*see Fig.* 14.3).

The Soft Tissue Profile

Various cephalometric assessments of the soft tissue profile have been proposed. It must be recognized that none of these can give guidance as to whether a particular face is attractive or not and such measurements are of very little diagnostic value. However, they may help in describing a patient's facial appearance. Perhaps the most useful of these is the Aesthetic Line which touches the tip of the nose and the tip of the chin. It has been maintained that the facial appearance is more likely to be pleasing when the lips lie close to this line. Another indicator is the naso-labial angle: ideally the naso-labial angle should be in the order of 110°. Too wide a naso-labial angle often gives a rather poor facial appearance. Orthodontic treatment, particularly with removable appliances, usually has a limited effect on the soft tissue profile and any major changes can usually be attributed to growth rather than to treatment.

Racial Variation

Note the norm figures given above have been derived from Caucasian groups and should not be applied to other racial groups.

Chapter 3

Soft Tissue Morphology and Behaviour

LIP FORM

The lips may be either competent or incompetent.
Competent lips. A lip seal can be maintained, with the mandible in the rest position, by minimal activity of the circumoral musculature (*Fig.* 3.1*a*). A patient with competent lips will normally obtain an anterior oral seal by lip contact. However, the lips may be habitually parted where, for example, the patient breathes through his mouth due to nasal obstruction or where prominent upper incisors prevent the lips from coming together.

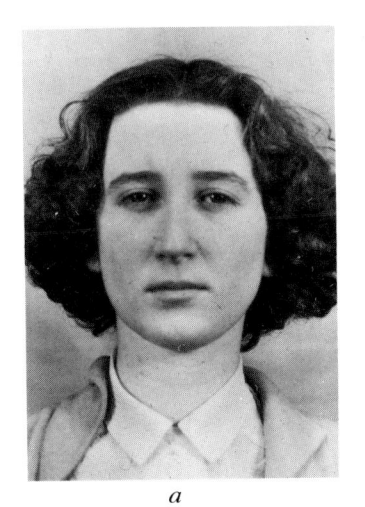

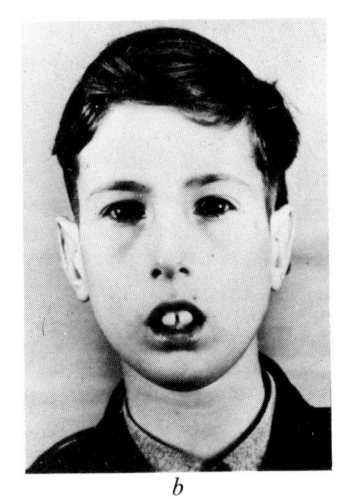

Fig. 3.1. *a*, Competent lips. *b*, Incompetent lips.

Incompetent lips. When the mandible is in the rest position and the circumoral muscles are at rest, the lips are parted (*Fig.* 3.1*b*). This is due to a disproportion between the lengths of the lips and the lower face height. The degree of incompetence varies: in some individuals a lip seal is maintained with only a slight contraction of the circumoral musculature; in others the lips are grossly incompetent and considerable muscular contraction is required to obtain a lip seal. Where the lips are grossly incompetent they will habitually be parted, but it must not be assumed that such an individual is a mouth breather; there will usually be an adaptive anterior oral seal between tongue and lower lip in addition to a posterior seal between the soft palate and dorsum of the tongue. In some cases where the lips are only mildly incompetent and there is a slight increase in overjet, the mandible will be habitually postured forwards so that a lip seal can be obtained with less total muscular effort.

It is important to recognize that incompetent lips cannot be made competent by exercise; exercise does not lengthen muscles. However, as a child matures, he is more likely to keep his lips together by a subconscious muscular effort provided that the degree of incompetence is not too great.

The orthodontic importance of lip incompetence is that the lower lip plays a major role in controlling the upper incisor position. The lower lip should cover the incisal third of the labial surface of the upper incisors. Where this is not the case because the lips are habitually parted, the upper incisors may be proclined. Before reduction of an overjet it is necessary to assess whether the patient is likely to maintain a lip seal after treatment. If this does not happen the overjet will increase again after appliances are discontinued.

Lip form is also of importance in determining the inclination of upper and lower incisors. Ballard suggested that it is the form of the lips which is of primary importance in determining the labiolingual inclination of the incisor teeth and that the tongue, unless it is abnormally large or small, acts to mould the teeth against the lips. This is an over-simplification and incisor position has, in turn, an effect on lip position. Thus there is a complex interplay between these factors. Clinically it is found that where the lips are full and everted both the upper and lower labial segments are often proclined (bimaxillary proclination), whereas in individuals with vertically positioned lips the upper and lower labial segments are often retroclined (bimaxillary retroclination).

THE TONGUE

The tongue adapts to the form of the oral cavity. In the infant the tongue lies between the gum pads in contact with the lips and cheeks. Feeding and swallowing take place with the tongue in this forward position. As teeth erupt oral function changes, and as mastication is established maturation from an infantile to an adult pattern of activity takes place gradually and is usually completed by the time the deciduous occlusion is established. However, in a number of children the infantile pattern of swallowing behaviour persists into the mixed dentition and this may influence the position of the incisor teeth.

Other variations in the first (oral) phase of swallowing may influence the position of the teeth. However, normal adult swallowing behaviour is described first.

After mastication the food is collected on the dorsum of the tongue. The teeth are then brought into light occlusion, there being contraction of the masseter and temporal muscles. This action closes the mouth cavity proper and separates it from the oral vestibule, forming as it were a solid box. Breathing stops for a moment. The tongue is placed against the palate and upper incisor teeth and a wave-like contraction then passes backwards carrying the food with it.

It should be noted that many minor variations of

swallowing behaviour are perfectly compatible with normal occlusion: for example, in idle swallowing of saliva the teeth are not usually brought into occlusion.

VARIATIONS IN SWALLOWING BEHAVIOUR
Persistent Infantile Swallowing Behaviour

Where the changeover to an adult pattern of swallowing does not take place at the usual time (during establishment of the deciduous occlusion) the incisor relationship may be affected: due to the forward position of the tongue in contact with the lower lip, the upper incisors become proclined and the overbite is incomplete. Usually this pattern will improve spontaneously before the child is 10 years of age. It could be argued that such patterns are frequently associated with incompetent lips or a thumb-sucking habit and this is merely a variation of the adaptive patterns of swallowing described below.

Adaptive Atypical Swallowing Behaviour Associated with:
Incompetent Lips

Where the lips are incompetent and habitually parted, an anterior oral seal may be obtained by contact between tongue and lower lip. This will be associated with proclination of the upper incisors and an incomplete overbite. The overbite is incomplete by only a small amount because if the teeth are brought into occlusion during swallowing, the tongue does not maintain contact with the lower lip.

If the upper incisors are retracted and the patient is then able to maintain a lip seal, a normal pattern of swallowing behaviour will return and so the result should be stable. However, if the lips are grossly incompetent so that an adaptive oral seal persists, the overjet will increase again after the appliances are discontinued.

Increase in Overjet

Where the overjet is large (perhaps associated with a Class II skeletal pattern), an adaptive oral seal between tongue and lower lip will be adopted (*see Fig.* 14.2, p. 140). The features are similar to those described above for incompetent lips.

Incomplete Overbite (or Anterior Open Bite)

If the overbite is incomplete, due for example to a thumb-sucking habit or an increased lower face height (*see* Chapter 10), the tongue will come forwards over the lower incisors during swallowing. As with all adaptive characteristics this will spontaneously revert to normal on correction of the malocclusion.

Primary Atypical Swallowing Behaviour

Rarely, there is an inborn atypical pattern of neuro-muscular activity so that the tongue is actively thrust forwards (endogenous tongue thrust) during swallowing (*Fig.* 3.2). This will produce an increase in overjet and a

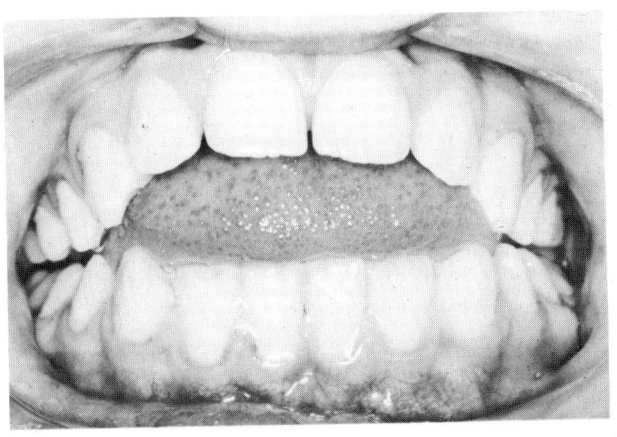

Fig. 3.2. A malocclusion associated with a primary atypical swallowing behaviour.

reduction in overbite. In these cases the overbite is quite markedly incomplete because during swallowing the posterior teeth are brought into occlusion while the tongue is thrust forwards over the lower incisors and against the palatal surface of the upper incisors. It is important to distinguish this unusual primary atypical pattern from the much more common adaptive variations in swallowing pattern, because in the former case correction of the malocclusion will not be stable. Clinically this distinction is not easy to make, but the following guidelines may be of help in recognizing primary atypical swallowing behaviour:

1. The tongue is thrust forwards more forcibly than with adaptive patterns and the amount of circumoral contraction seems to be greater than would have been expected from the degree of lip incompetence.

2. The incompleteness of overbite is greater than is found with the adaptive swallowing patterns associated with lip incompetence or a large overjet (*Fig.* 3.2). However, it is important to rule out thumb-sucking habits or skeletal factors because they can be associated with similar malocclusions.

3. Sometimes these patients exhibit lisps or other speech defects. However, this is not an infallible guide and many children with speech defects have normal occlusions.

CONCLUSION

The teeth are in a position of balance determined by the interaction between the soft tissues, the jaw relationship and occlusal forces. If the position of the teeth is to be changed and remain stable, another position of balance must be sought. Generally, and provided that the skeletal malrelationship is not severe, the lower arch is a good guide to a position of stability of the upper arch. However, where there are marked variations of soft tissue pattern or behaviour this may not be so. These variations are not common but it is important to recognize them when they do occur and to take this into account in planning treatment.

Chapter 4

Mandibular Positions and Paths of Closure

The fundamental position of the mandible is the rest position which is determined by the resting length of the muscles acting on it. By definition, the rest position of the mandible is that position in which the muscles acting on it exhibit minimal activity as measured electromyographically. The rest position is not influenced by the position of the teeth: the teeth and alveolar processes grow up from their respective dental bases and the occlusal level is established a few millimetres short of the rest position. In this position, there is a balance between the forces of eruption of the teeth and the forces of muscular contraction. The interocclusal clearance when the mandible is in the rest position is the freeway space.

Centric relation is defined as those positions of the mandible in which the condyles are in retruded unstrained positions in the glenoid fossae. The rest position is, and the position of maximal occlusion should be, a position of centric relation and so the path of closure between these two positions should be a simple hinge movement of the mandible about an axis just below the condylar heads.

In some patients with Class II division 1 incisor relationships the mandible may be habitually postured downward and forward from the rest position, possibly to facilitate a lip seal or for aesthetic reasons. In these circumstances the path of closure of the mandible will be upwards and backwards into the occlusal position, i.e. there will be a deviation of the mandible on closure.

Although the position of maximal occlusion should be a position of centric relation, in a number of patients, due to occlusal interferences (premature contacts), the mandible is displaced during its path of closure from the rest to the occlusal position. Displacements may be lateral (e.g. if there is a unilateral crossbite, p. 133), anterior (e.g. if there are instanding incisors, p. 158), or rarely posterior (e.g. if there has been loss of posterior teeth and there is a Class II division 2 incisor relationship).

It is important to recognize and distinguish between deviations and displacements of the mandible during closure from the rest position into occlusion. Deviations are important because they are associated with habit postures. These must be recognized at diagnosis because if the dental base relationship is assessed when the mandible is in the habit posture a misleading impression of the skeletal pattern will be given; and the patient will lose the habit posture when the incisor relationship is changed during treatment. However, habit postures do not seem to be associated with pain or dysfunction.

Displacements, in contrast with deviations, are associated with occlusal dysfunction, and in the long term may give rise to muscle or joint pain. The factor responsible for the displacement should be corrected as early as possible. Patients with a sagittal displacement of the mandible may exhibit overclosure. This is sometimes found where there is a mild Class III incisor relationship with an overbite. The patient can obtain an edge-to-edge incisor relationship but with the posterior teeth out of occlusion. The slight forward displacement to avoid the premature contact of the incisors is associated with overclosure. On correction of the incisor relationship it will be found that the posterior teeth do not meet, but they will usually erupt into occlusion.

Chapter 5

Development of Normal Occlusion

AT BIRTH

At birth the maxillary and mandibular gum pads have 20 segmented elevations corresponding to the unerupted deciduous teeth. The elevations for the second deciduous molars are poorly defined at birth and are not properly present until the age of 5 months. The groove that marks the distal margin of the canine segment continues into the buccal sulcus and is called the 'lateral sulcus'.

The upper arch is horseshoe-shaped and the vault of the palate is very shallow. The alveolar part is separated on its palatal side from the hard palate by a continuous horizontal groove known as the 'dental or gingival groove'. The lower arch is U-shaped and the gum pad anteriorly is slightly everted labially.

With the mandible in its physiological rest position the gum pads are apart, with the tongue filling the space between them and projecting against the lips anteriorly, the lower lip forming the principal boundary to the front of the oral cavity. The upper lip appears to be very short at this age.

The gum pads rarely come into occlusion. The maxillary gum pad overlaps the mandibular both buccally and labially, corresponding to the ultimate occlusal relationship of the teeth (*Fig.* 5.1). The gum pads at birth are not sufficiently wide to accommodate the developing incisors which are crowded and rotated in their crypts, the lateral being rotated distolingually. But during the first year of life they grow rapidly, especially laterally. This ultimately permits incisors to erupt in good alignment, helped by pressure from the tongue and lips.

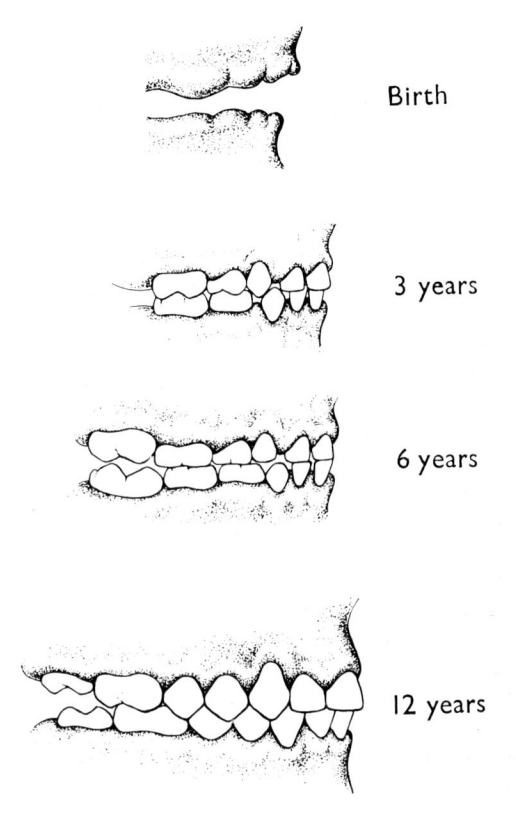

Fig. 5.1. Stages in the development of normal occlusion.

THE DECIDUOUS DENTITION (*Table* 5.1)

Eruption of the lower central incisors begins at about 6 months of age. It should be recognized that the timing of eruption is very variable and a range of 6 months on either side of the representative figures given in *Table* 5.1 is commonplace. Usually by the age of $2\frac{1}{2}$ years all the deciduous teeth have erupted (*Fig.* 5.1).

Table 5.1. Typical ages of eruption and mesiodistal widths of the deciduous teeth

	Time of eruption (months)	Mesiodistal width (mm)
Maxillary teeth		
Central incisor	8	6·5
Lateral incisor	9	5·0
Canine	18	6·5
First molar	14	7·0
Second molar	24	8·5
Mandibular teeth		
Central incisor	6	4·0
Lateral incisor	7	4·5
Canine	16	5·5
First molar	12	8·0
Second molar	20	9·5

Notes:
1. Eruption times vary considerably. Up to 6 months earlier or later than the times given is not unusual.
2. Mesiodistal widths vary by up to 20% on either side of the figures given.
3. Calcification of the deciduous teeth begins between 4 and 6 months *in utero*.
4. Root formation is complete between 12 and 18 months after eruption.

Points to Notice at 2½ Years

1. The incisors are more vertical than their permanent successors and they are often spaced.
2. There may be spacings distal to the lower canines and mesial to the upper canines (the so-called 'primate spacings').
3. The second deciduous molars are flush distally.

Changes in the Deciduous Occlusion (between 2½ and 5½ Years)

1. In some children there is an increase in spacing of the incisors associated with an increase in arch width.

2. Provided that there has been occlusal attrition of the teeth, the lower arch will often move forwards relative to the upper to establish an edge-to-edge incisor occlusion. This is probably due to a change in jaw relationship with the mandible growing forwards relative to the maxilla.

THE MIXED DENTITION (*Table* 5.2)

At the age of 6 years permanent teeth, usually the first molars or lower central incisors, start to erupt. As in the case of the deciduous teeth, eruption times and the order of eruption are very variable and a range of 18 months on either side of the figures given in *Table* 5.2 is not unusual.

The Permanent Incisors

The permanent incisors develop lingual to the roots of the deciduous incisors (*Fig.* 5.2). Space for these teeth, which are larger than their deciduous predecessors, is provided by:

1. Utilization of existing spacing between the deciduous incisors.

2. An increase in intercanine width takes place during the eruption of the incisors.

3. The upper permanent incisors are more proclined and thus form a larger arch than the deciduous incisors.

Notes:

a. If the deciduous incisor root is not resorbed normally, the permanent incisor may be deflected lingually.

b. The upper lateral incisors in their developmental position are overlapped by the central incisors (*Fig.* 5.2). They escape as the central incisors erupt. However, if there is not sufficient growth in arch width they may be trapped in this palatal position.

c. When the upper incisors erupt they are frequently

Table 5.2. Typical ages of eruption and mesiodistal widths of the permanent teeth

	Time of eruption (years)	Mesiodistal width (mm)
Maxillary teeth		
Central incisor	7·5	8·5
Lateral incisor	8·5	6·5
Canine	11·5	8·0
First premolar	10·0	7·0
Second premolar	11·0	6·5
First molar	6·0	10·0
Second molar	12·0	9·5
Mandibular teeth		
Central incisor	6·5	5·5
Lateral incisor	7·5	6·0
Canine	10·0	7·0
First premolar	10·5	7·0
Second premolar	11·0	7·0
First molar	6·0	11·0
Second molar	12·0	10·5

Notes:
1. The figures given both for eruption times and for mesiodistal widths commonly vary by up to 20% on either side of the figures given.
2. Calcification dates are variable but the permanent teeth have usually started to calcify as follows:

At birth $\dfrac{/6}{/6}$

By 6 months $\dfrac{/1\ 3}{/123}$

By 2 years $\dfrac{/24}{/\ 4}$

By 4 years $\dfrac{/5\ 7}{/5\ 7}$

Between 8 and 14 years $\dfrac{/8}{/8}$

3. Root formation is normally completed 2–3 years after eruption.

DEVELOPMENT OF NORMAL OCCLUSION 41

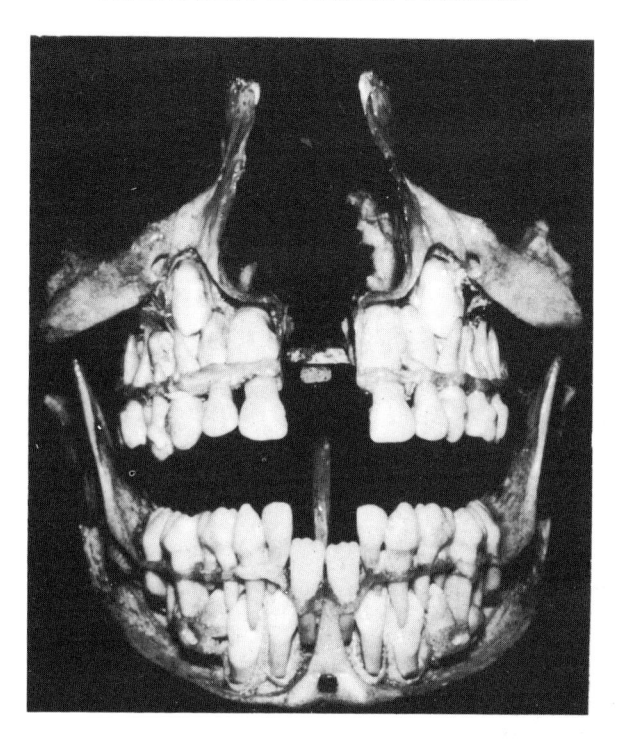

Fig. 5.2. Developmental positions of the permanent incisors. Note that the permanent incisors develop lingual to the roots of the deciduous incisors and that the upper lateral incisors are overlapped by the central incisors and canines.

distally inclined so that there is a median diastema (*Fig.* 5.3). This is the 'ugly duckling' stage and is due to the incisor roots being crowded mesially by the permanent canine crowns. When the permanent canines erupt the median diastema (physiological spacing) will usually close. This natural developmental stage should not be mistaken for a malocclusion and treatment must not be undertaken to close the diastema before the permanent canines erupt.

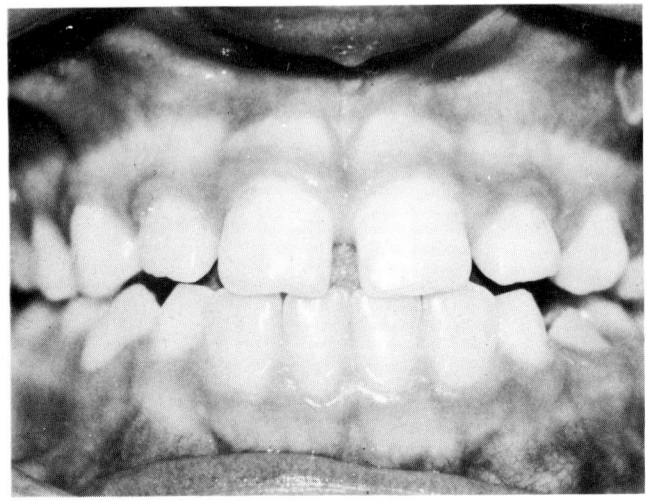

Fig. 5.3. The 'ugly duckling' stage.

The Permanent Canines and Premolars

Although the permanent canines are wider than their predecessors, the premolars, particularly the second premolars, are narrower than the deciduous molars. Thus the combined mesiodistal width of the permanent canines and premolars is usually less than that of the deciduous canines and molars. The surplus space, the leeway space, is greater in the lower arch and is taken up by mesial drift of the first permanent molars.

The Permanent Molars

These are guided into a cusp-to-cusp relationship by the distal surfaces of the second deciduous molars (*Fig.* 5.1). This is a normal occlusal relationship in the mixed dentition. The lower molar may erupt slightly in advance of the upper if the lower arch has moved forwards relative to the upper in the deciduous dentition (*see* p. 39). When the second deciduous molars are shed the greater leeway space in the lower arch allows the lower first permanent molars to move forwards into a correct cuspal relationship with the upper (*Fig.* 5.1). The second permanent molars should be guided directly into occlusion by the first permanent molars.

The upper permanent molars develop in the maxillary tuberosity with their occlusal surfaces facing distally and buccally as well as occlusally. Posterior growth in maxillary length is necessary to allow them to rotate forwards and downwards into the line of the arch. The mandibular molars develop under the anterior border of the ascending ramus of the mandible. Growth in mandibular length, which involves resorption on the anterior margin of the ascending ramus, is necessary if the tooth is to have room to erupt.

THE PERMANENT DENTITION

Without going into exact details of the positions of each tooth, the following points should be noted (*Fig.* 5.1).

1. The mandibular teeth are set one inclined plane in advance of the maxillary teeth. This is so because the mandibular central incisor is smaller mesiodistally than the maxillary central incisor.

2. The maxillary teeth are half a cusp to the buccal of the mandibular teeth (i.e. they are not cusp-to-cusp).

3. Angle stated that the mesiobuccal cusp of the upper first permanent molar occludes with the anterior buccal groove of the lower first permanent molar. In fact, if the upper second premolar is wide, this is too far forward. This can be checked by examining the distobuccal cusp of the first permanent molar which should occlude in the embrasure between the lower first and second permanent molars.

4. The upper permanent canine occludes in the embrasure between the lower permanent canine and first premolar.

5. The lower incisor edges occlude with the cingulum plateau of the upper incisors (*see Fig.* 6.5*a*, p. 52). Provided that the incisor inclinations are average this gives a normal overbite of about one-third of the height of the lower incisor crowns and an overjet of about 2 mm.

Changes in the Permanent Occlusion

Certain natural changes in the permanent occlusion are found in some cases:

An Increase in Incisor Crowding

This may be associated with mandibular growth rotations and corresponding dento-alveolar adaptation as described on pp. 13–14.

It has also been suggested that mesial drift of buccal teeth may contribute to this late crowding. Mesial drift is observed when the continuity of the arch is broken by extraction of teeth but the cause is not understood. The following explanations have been offered:

1. It is a natural growth tendency in the human.

2. Crowded teeth, particularly third molars, exert a forward pressure on the other teeth. It should be noted, however, that mesial drift occurs even where third molars are developmentally absent.

3. The anterior component of force: this arises because the upper and lower teeth are slightly mesially inclined. Vertical occlusal loading produces an intrusive force and a small anterior component of force which could be responsible for mesial drift. However, the evidence in support of this theory is insubstantial.

Changes in Arch Relationship in the Permanent Occlusion

With growth there is a tendency for the mandible to grow slightly further forward than the maxilla (*see* Chapter 2). In normal occlusion with good intercuspation of the teeth there will usually be no appreciable occlusal change. However, if there are marked changes in jaw relationships corresponding occlusal changes will be found.

Chapter 6

Malocclusion

A malocclusion is defined as an irregularity of teeth beyond the accepted range of normal. Thus malocclusions are for the most part variations around the normal and are a representation of biological variability. Biological variation is expressed elsewhere in the body but minor irregularities are more readily noticed and recorded in the dentition and occlusion and so have attracted greater attention and associated demands for treatment. The majority of malocclusions are primarily of hereditary causation although some environmental factors, such as unplanned extraction of teeth, are of importance.

There is evidence that the prevalence of malocclusion is increasing, particularly in developed communities. This increase may in part reflect an underlying evolutionary trend towards shorter jaws and fewer teeth, but it is probably largely the result of an increase in the genetic variability of these populations brought about by intermixture of racial groups. It has been proposed by Begg that one reason for the increase in the prevalence of crowding is that there is now little approximal or occlusal attrition of the teeth. In primitive people living on a coarse diet an appreciable reduction in the mesiodistal widths of erupted teeth occurs due to attrition. This loss of tooth substance, which can amount to several millimetres in each quadrant, would reduce any crowding.

Malocclusions may be associated with one or more of the following: (1) malposition of individual teeth; (2) malrelationship of the dental arches.

MALPOSITION OF INDIVIDUAL TEETH

A tooth may occupy a position other than normal by being:

1. Tilted or inclined: the apex is normally placed but the crown is incorrectly positioned.
2. Displaced: both apex and crown are incorrectly positioned.
3. Rotated: the tooth is rotated around its long axis.
4. In infra-occlusion: the tooth has not reached the occlusal level.
5. In supra-occlusion: the tooth has erupted past the occlusal level.
6. Transposed: two teeth have reversed their positions, for example an upper canine and first premolar.

Teeth which are tilted or displaced are described according to the direction of the malposition: for example, an incisor may be labially inclined (or proclined), lingually inclined (or retroclined), mesially inclined, or distally inclined. Similar terms apply to displacements. Rotations are described by the approximal surface which is furthest from the line of the arch and the direction in which it faces: for example, a rotated upper incisor is described as mesiolabially rotated if the mesial aspect is out of the line of the arch while a similar rotation would be described as distopalatal if the distal aspect were palatally positioned.

MALRELATIONSHIPS OF THE DENTAL ARCHES

Malrelationships of the arches may occur in any of the three planes of space: antero-posterior, vertical or transverse. The aetiology and treatment of vertical and transverse malrelationships are dealt with in Chapter 12. The classifications of malocclusion described in this text are based on antero-posterior relationships as described below. The aetiology and treatment of these malrelationships are dealt with in Chapters 13–16.

CLASSIFICATION OF MALOCCLUSION

For convenience of description, it is useful to have some classification which will divide up the wide range of malocclusions into a small number of groups. Many classifications have been proposed but the one which is universally recognized is Angle's classification which is based on arch relationship in the sagittal plane. The key relationship in Angle's classification is that of the first permanent molars: in normal occlusions, the anterior buccal groove of the lower first permanent molar should occlude with the anterior buccal cusp of the upper first permanent molar (*see Fig.* 1.1, p. 2). If the first molars have drifted this must be allowed for before the occlusion is classified.

Angle's Classification

Class I. Malocclusions in which the lower first permanent molar is within one half cusp width of its correct relationship to the upper first permanent molar (*Fig.* 6.1). This arch relationship is sometimes known as 'neutro-occlusion'.

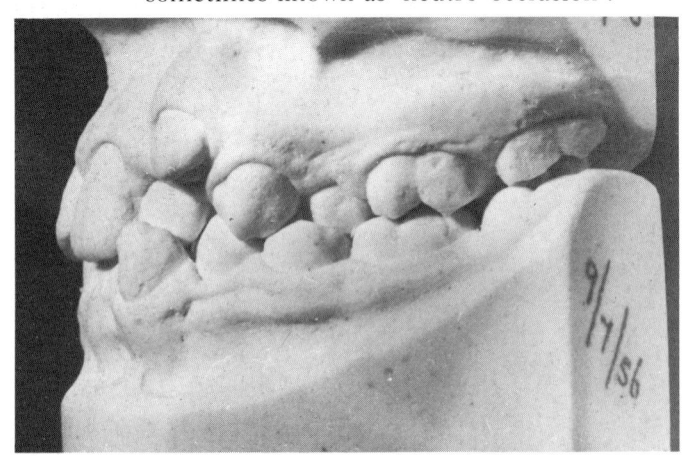

Fig. 6.1. An Angle's Class I malocclusion.

Class II. The lower arch is at least one-half cusp width posterior to the correct relationship with the upper arch, judged by the first molar relationship (*Figs.* 6.2 and 6.3). This arch relationship is sometimes known as 'disto-occlusion'.

Class II is divided according to the inclination of the upper central incisors:

Division 1. The upper central incisors are proclined or of average inclination so that there is an increase in overjet (*Fig.* 6.2).

Division 2. The upper central incisors are retroclined (*Fig.* 6.3) (less than 105° to the maxillary plane). The overjet is usually average but may be a little increased. Sometimes the upper lateral incisors are proclined, mesially inclined and mesiolabially rotated.

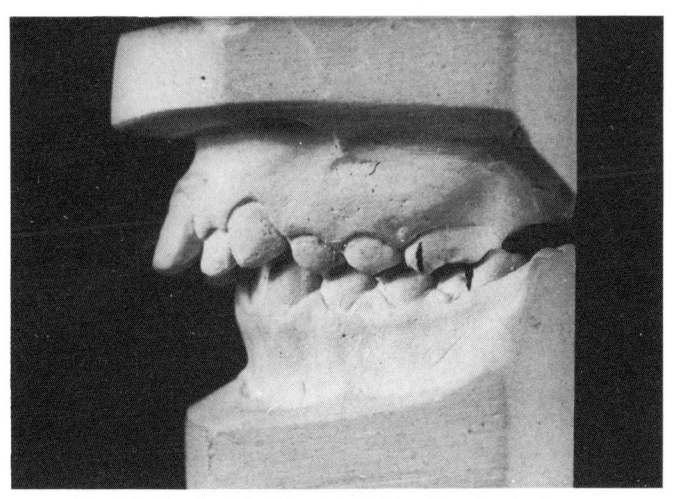

Fig. 6.2. An Angle's Class II division 1 malocclusion.

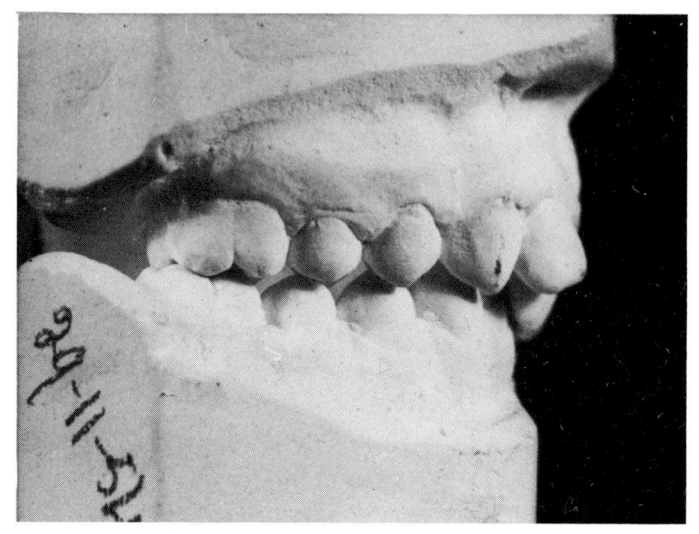

Fig. 6.3. An Angle's Class II division 2 malocclusion.

Class III. The lower arch is at least one-half cusp width too far forward in relation to the upper arch, judged by the first permanent molar relationship (*Fig.* 6.4). This arch relationship is sometimes known as 'mesio-occlusion'.

A number of problems may be encountered in classifying a particular malocclusion according to Angle.

a. The first permanent molars may have been extracted or they may have drifted following early loss of deciduous molar teeth (*Fig.* 6.4). Where the first molars have drifted forwards as a result of early loss, this should be allowed for before classification. This is not always simple and it is well worthwhile looking at the general features of the occlusion and in particular at the permanent canine relationship. The upper permanent canine should occlude into the embrasure between the lower canine and first premolar. This relationship should match the first permanent molar relationship: in Class II cases the embrasure

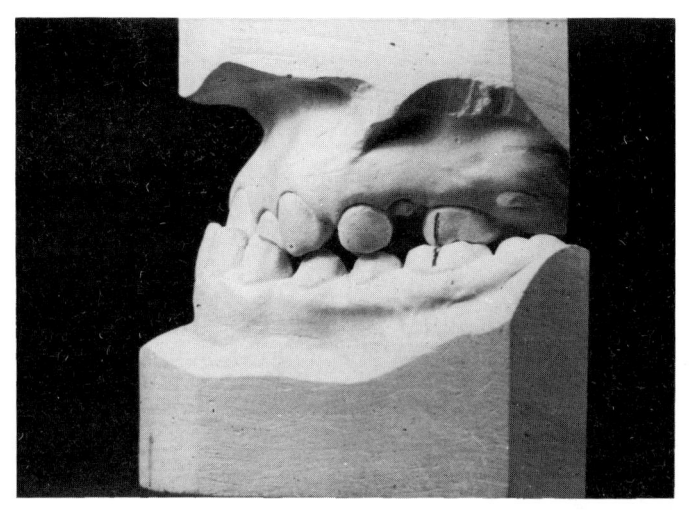

Fig. 6.4. An Angle's Class III malocclusion. Note that the upper first permanent molar has drifted forwards following early loss of a deciduous molar. This must be allowed for before classifying the malocclusion.

between the lower canine and first premolar will be distal to the cusp of the upper canine where, as in Class III cases, it will be too far forwards. In general, if the molar and canine relationship match one another the classification can be affirmed with reasonable confidence; but if they do not, care must be taken and classification may have to be undertaken on the general features of the occlusion.

b. The occlusion may differ between sides. Angle allowed for this by describing subdivisions of Class II and Class III where one side was in a normal relationship. However, it is probably more useful to classify the occlusion according to its general features.

c. It can be difficult to know where to draw the dividing line between Class I and the other classes. Here again, the final decision must rest on the general features of the occlusion.

Angle considered that the first permanent molars had

constant developmental relationships to their respective jaws so that, by classifying the occlusion, the skeletal pattern could also be assessed. It must be emphasized that this assumption is *not* correct and that the developmental positions of the teeth on the jaws may vary. Thus the occlusal classification and skeletal classification are not necessarily coincident.

Incisor Classification

The incisor relationship does not always match the buccal segment relationship. As much orthodontic treatment is focused on correction of incisor malrelationships, it is helpful to have a classification of incisor relationships (*Fig.* 6.5). The terms used are the same but this is *not* Angle's classification. The incisor classification may be found to be more useful in clinical practice than is Angle's classification.

Class I. The lower incisor edges occlude with or lie immediately below the cingulum plateau (middle part of the palatal surface) of the upper central incisors (*Fig.* 6.5*a*).

Class II. The lower incisor edges lie posterior to the cingulum plateau of the upper incisors.

There are two divisions to Class II malocclusion:

Division 1. The upper central incisors are proclined or of average inclination and there is an increase in overjet (*Fig.* 6.5*b*).

Division 2. The upper central incisors are retroclined (less than 105° to the maxillary plane). The overjet is usually average but may be increased (*Fig.* 6.5*c*).

Class III. The lower incisor edges lie anterior to the cingulum plateau of the upper incisors (*Fig.* 6.5*d*). The overjet is reduced or reversed.

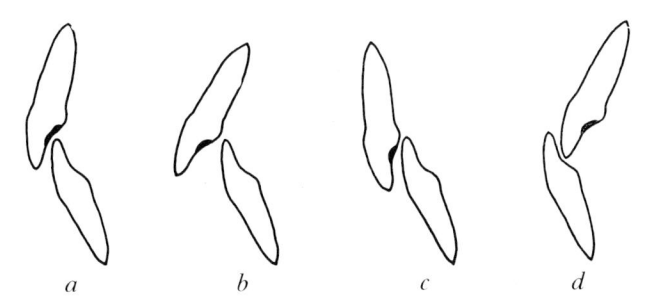

Fig. 6.5. Incisor classification: *a*, Class I; *b*, Class II division 1; *c*, Class II division 2; *d*, Class III.

THE AETIOLOGY OF MALOCCLUSION

For convenience of discussion, the causes of malocclusion can broadly be divided into general factors and local factors.

General factors are discussed in detail in the relevant chapters and include variations in skeletal relationship (Chapter 2), disproportion between tooth size and arch size resulting in crowding or spacing (Chapter 11) and soft tissue factors (Chapter 3).

Malocclusions are also associated with a number of genetic and developmental disorders such as Down's syndrome (mongolism), hypothyroidism (cretinism), cleidocranial dysostosis and many other relatively uncommon syndromes. These are not discussed in this text. However, because of their dental importance and comparative frequency the malocclusions associated with cleft palate are described in Chapter 20.

Local factors are essentially habits and anomalies in the number, form and developmental positions of the teeth. In spite of their classification as local factors, their effects may be quite extensive. Local factors may coexist with one another and with any of the general factors mentioned above. They will be discussed in Chapter 10.

Chapter 7

Tissue Changes with Tooth Movement

The classic experiments on tissue changes following orthodontic tooth movements were carried out by Sandstedt (1905), by Oppenheim, first on monkeys (1911) and ultimately on humans (1931), and by Reitan (1951).

Normal alveolar bone. This consists of a layer of lamellated compact bone adjacent to the periodontal membrane (lamina dura) and oral mucosa with cancellous or spongy bone in between these two compact layers. The lamellae of the compact bone are parallel to the long axis of the tooth. Labially and buccally to the teeth the bone is almost entirely compact.

Types of Tooth Movement

Tipping (Fig. 7.1)

This is produced by removable orthodontic appliances. With light forces the fulcrum is about 40% of the length of the root from the apex.

Bodily Movement and Rotation

These are not practicable with removable appliances. However, most fixed appliances are capable of producing bodily tooth movements and rotations.

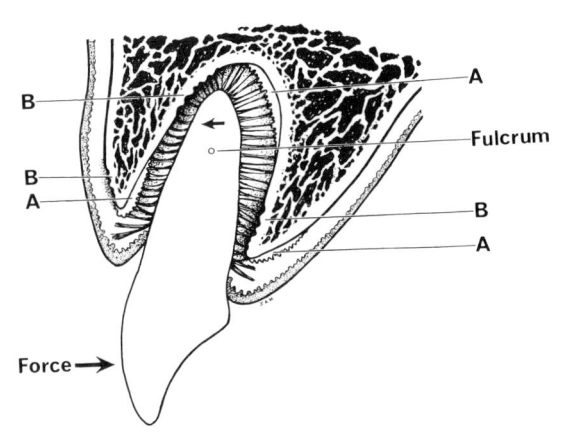

Fig. 7.1. The effects of a tipping force. A, Areas of bone deposition. B, Areas of bone resorption.

Depression and Elongation

The force distribution within the periodontal ligament depends on the nature of the tooth movement. With tipping movements, areas of maximal pressure and tension are set up at the apical and cervical regions of the root, whereas with bodily movements the force is distributed reasonably evenly along the root axis.

Tissue Changes

The tissue changes produced depend principally on the values and duration of the forces used. Different regions of the periodontal ligament may show different types of tissue reaction at the one time depending on the force values within the periodontium at that particular point. Within the first 24 hours after the application of the force, the tooth moves some way through the periodontal space, setting up areas of tension and compression within the periodontium.

Areas of Pressure

Light forces (e.g. 30 g (1 oz) per single-rooted tooth for tipping movement). The periodontal ligament is compressed but not crushed. The blood vessels are still patent. Within 24–48 hours osteoclasts appear along the bone surface and direct bone resorption proceeds. Within the cancellous spaces, deposition of osteoid takes place (*Fig. 7.1*).

Heavy forces. The periodontal ligament is crushed between the tooth and the socket wall. The blood vessels are occluded and the periodontal ligament becomes acellular and hyaline in appearance. The osteocytes of the underlying bone die. These hyalinized areas are often fairly localized, and adjacent to them and within the cancellous spaces of the underlying bone osteoclasts appear. In this manner the hyalinized area is removed by undermining resorption and the tooth will eventually move. If the range of action of the spring has been large, the force applied will still be excessive and further areas of hyalinization will appear.

Areas of Tension

Initially there is a proliferation of fibroblasts and pre-osteoblasts and the periodontal fibres are elongated. Osteoid tissue is deposited along the bone surface in spicules, lying in the direction of the stretched periodontal fibres. This osteoid tissue is progressively replaced by bundle bone.

Where heavy forces have been used the periodontal fibres on the tension side may be torn and blood vessels ruptured. When the tooth is being moved labially or palatally, modelling resorption and deposition on the external alveolar surface, particularly in the marginal region, will maintain the thickness and contour of the alveolar plates.

Retention

During the period of retention further tissue changes take place. In the tension areas the remaining osteoid is replaced by bundle bone and the bundle bone is reorganized to form lamellated bone with Haversian systems. In the regions of pressure the osteoclasts remain for up to 2 weeks. Osteoid is deposited over the areas of resorption and, in due course, this is replaced by bundle bone and ultimately by mature lamellated bone.

The periodontal fibres also become reorganized during the retention period. Most of these changes are completed within 6 months. However, reorganization is much slower after certain tooth movements, e.g. after rotations, the trans-septal and free gingival fibres remain displaced for a considerable time. It is possible that the failure of re-adaptation of these fibres contributes towards relapse of such tooth movements. For this reason, surgical section or pericision (*Fig.* 7.2) of these fibres may be undertaken following tooth alignment. This does not always eliminate relapse but appears to be effective in reducing the relapse tendency provided that it is correctly done. The tooth

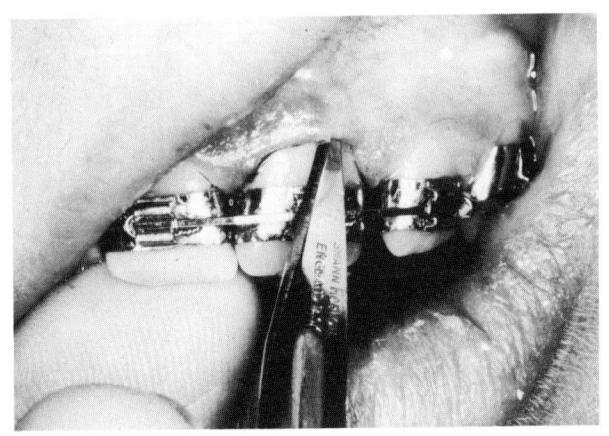

Fig. 7.2. Pericision. The free gingival fibres and trans-septal fibres are severed.

should then be retained in the conventional manner for about 6 months.

Forces used. The threshold value below which tooth movement will not occur is probably very low. For tipping movements a very light force should be applied initially and this can be increased to about 30 g (1 oz) for a single-rooted tooth. The force applied should be proportional to the root area and correspondingly heavier forces may be applied to molar teeth.

Heavier forces may also be used for bodily tooth movement as the force is more evenly distributed throughout the periodontal ligament.

The Rate of Tooth Movement

About 1 mm per month may be regarded as an acceptable rate of tooth movement. Various factors affect the rate of tooth movement.

The Force Applied

Both light and heavy forces will result in orthodontic tooth movement. However, it is generally felt that if light forces are used, minimizing hyalinization of the periodontal ligament, the rate of tooth movement will be greater.

Age

In the adult, the periodontal ligament is much less cellular than in the child. In addition, the alveolar bone in children is less dense than in older patients. This means that, in general, tooth movement in the adult will be slower.

Individual Variations

There is considerable individual variation in the response to orthodontic forces. This is at least in part dependent on the density of the alveolar bone. In some individuals the alveolar bone is loose and cancellous with large marrow spaces, whereas in others it is dense lamellated bone with few marrow spaces. Tooth movement will be much slower in the latter.

Harmful Effects of Orthodontic Tooth Movement

Pulp Death

This is not common but can result from the application of heavy forces, particularly if the apex of the tooth is closed.

Root Resorption

Minor areas of resorption of cementum on the lateral aspects of the root may be seen during orthodontic tooth movement. These are not important and are repaired by cementum. Much more serious is the apical resorption sometimes seen, particularly when teeth have been moved bodily over long distances by fixed appliances. This can be extensive and little can be done. If such root resorption is observed during treatment the tooth movement should be stopped for some months to allow repair by secondary cementum and then, if absolutely necessary, tooth movement may be very carefully recommenced. It is important to recognize that root resorption is not uncommon in patients who have not received orthodontic treatment. For this reason all teeth to be moved should be radiographed prior to treatment. If root resorption is observed one should be very cautious about undertaking treatment.

GENERAL CONCLUSIONS

It is generally thought that only light forces should be used for orthodontic tooth movement. Both vital and non-vital teeth can be moved.

Orthodontic movement is possible only because cementum is more resistant to resorption than bone. Some writers recommend intermittent pressure, some constant pressure. Here again, little difference exists between the two clinically.

When excessive force is used it is very likely that the anchor teeth may move, the amount of force applied to them being ideal for this, whereas the tooth that it is desired to move will not move because the force is too strong.

Chapter 8

Principles and Components of Removable Appliances

Removable appliances are orthodontic devices which can be taken out by the patient for cleaning and which may be designed to apply forces to the teeth by means of springs, screws and other mechanical components. Myofunctional appliances, which depend for their action on the orofacial musculature, are described in Chapter 18.

Removable appliance components are discussed under the following headings: active component; retention; anchorage; baseplate.

ACTIVE COMPONENT

The active component of a removable appliance is the means by which forces are applied to the teeth to bring about the required movement. These mechanisms include springs (and bows), screws and elastics.

Springs are made from hard stainless steel wire. The simplest spring is the cantilever (*Fig.* 8.1*a*). The factors affecting the force (F) applied by this spring are given by the expression:

$$F \propto dr^4/l^3,$$

i.e. the force is directly proportioned to the deflection (d), to the fourth power of the radius (r) and inversely proportional to the cube of the length (l). Thus small variations in the length and particularly in the diameter of the wire will have major effects on the spring characteristics.

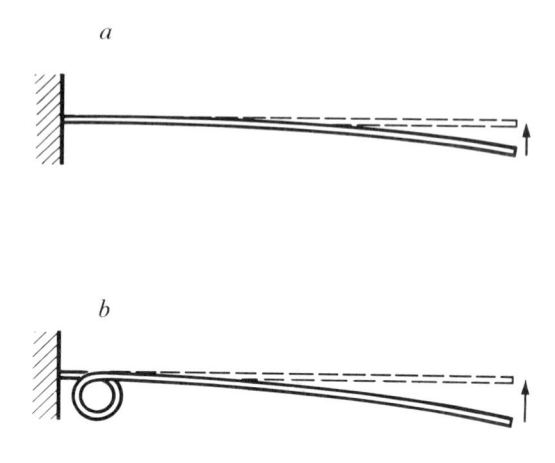

Fig. 8.1. *a*, A simple cantilever. *b*, The incorporation of a coil increases the deflection of the spring for a given load. Note that the coil should unwind as the tooth moves.

A well designed spring should be flexible in the direction of activation but stiff in other directions. The ratio of these is the stability ratio. A low stability ratio indicates that the spring is liable to be unstable and will be difficult to adjust.

It is usually appropriate to apply a force as light as possible for a given deflection and so the wire should be made as long as possible within the confines of the oral cavity and as thin as is consistent with adequate strength. The effective length of the spring may be increased by incorporating a coil (*Fig.* 8.1*b*).

For maximal stored energy (i.e. resilience) the coil should unwind as the force is dissipated (*Fig.* 8.1*b*). This is not always possible with buccal springs. For palatal springs wire of 0·5 mm diameter may be used but self-supporting buccal springs (*see Fig.* 9.3) should be 0·7 mm in diameter. The spring must be carefully designed so that

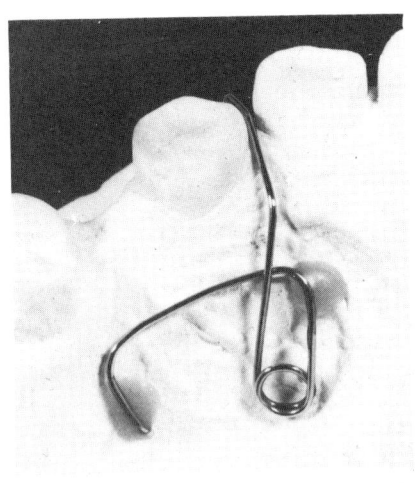

Fig. 8.2. A palatal spring with a guard. This spring is positioned so that the tooth will be moved in the line of the arch: the tooth will move perpendicular to the tangent to the surface at the point of contact with the spring.

the tooth will move in the direction intended. The direction of movement is perpendicular to the tangent to the tooth surface at the point of contact of the spring (*Fig.* 8.2). It is very common to find that palatal springs are placed too far back so that the resultant force is buccally directed. Palatal finger springs are readily distorted and should be protected either by being boxed within a recess of the base plate or guarded by a length of wire or preferably both (*see Fig.* 9.2). The free action of the spring must not be impeded by the box or guards. When adjusting a spring, it is important not to bend it where it emerges from the baseplate, otherwise it will fracture in use. Adjustments should be made in the free arm of the spring, taking care that the direction of action is correct. The force applied to a single-rooted tooth should be in the region of 30 g (1 oz). With a typical palatal spring used to retract a canine, an adjustment of about 3 mm (less than one-half of the mesiodistal width of the tooth) will be appropriate. Self-supporting buccal springs are much more rigid and activation should be correspondingly small (1–2 mm in the case of a typical buccal spring for canine retraction). Their stability ratio is poor. Supported buccal retractors (*see Fig.* 9.3*b*) have a better stability ratio and are more satisfactory in use.

Labial bows (*see Fig.* 9.4) are mechanically more complex than springs and their flexibility in the horizontal plane depends to a great extent on the height of any vertical loops incorporated in them. Most unsupported bows are made from 0·7 mm diameter wire but have a poor stability ratio. Supported bows, such as the Robert's retractor (*see Fig.* 9.8), are made from 0·5 mm diameter wire. This bow made from thinner wire is very much more flexible, while the stability ratio is favourable.

Screws may be designed to act directly on the teeth or, by separating two parts of the baseplate, to apply forces to the teeth through the baseplate (*see Fig.* 9.11). A screw applies a large intermittent force to the teeth. In most cases screws should be activated, by the patient, one-quarter turn each week. This opens the screw by about 0·2 mm. Thus the tooth movement is small and the periodontal ligament is not crushed. As the optimal rate of tooth movement is about 1 mm a month, weekly activation of the screw is usually appropriate. Screws have the disadvantages that, compared with springs, they are bulky and expensive. However, they are very useful in certain situations.

Elastics are commonly used for intermaxillary traction with fixed appliances and for extra-oral traction. They are not commonly used as the active component of a removable appliance because they tend to ride up the teeth and damage the gingival tissues (*Fig.* 8.3). It is very important that an elastic should *not* be attached directly to an individual tooth because it may work its way up to the gingival tissues and cause severe trauma.

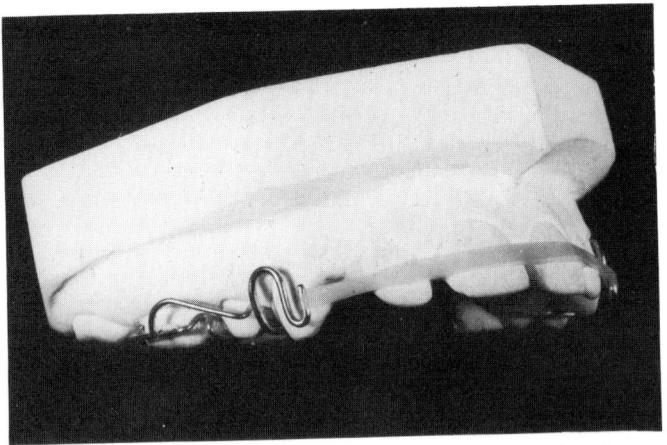

Fig. 8.3. The retraction of upper incisors with a latex elastic. *Note*: This is not recommended because the elastic tends to slip up the tooth surface and damage the gingivae.

RETENTION

Retention is the means by which the appliance resists displacement. In removable appliances retention is provided by clasps and labial bows. Retention must be adequate but an excessive number of clasps should be avoided. If extra-oral traction is to be used, retention must be good. An appliance which is not retentive will be uncomfortable for the patient and will often not be worn.

The major retention component of modern removable appliances is the Adams' clasp. This is simple to construct using universal pliers and is very efficient. It makes use of the undercuts on the mesiobuccal and distobuccal aspect of the teeth (*Fig.* 8.4a). (For details of construction and variations of design *see* Adams, 1970.) For satisfactory use it is important that these clasps are correctly made. Badly made clasps are not retentive and are difficult to adjust clinically.

Fitted labial bows (*see Fig.* 9.18) may be used to improve

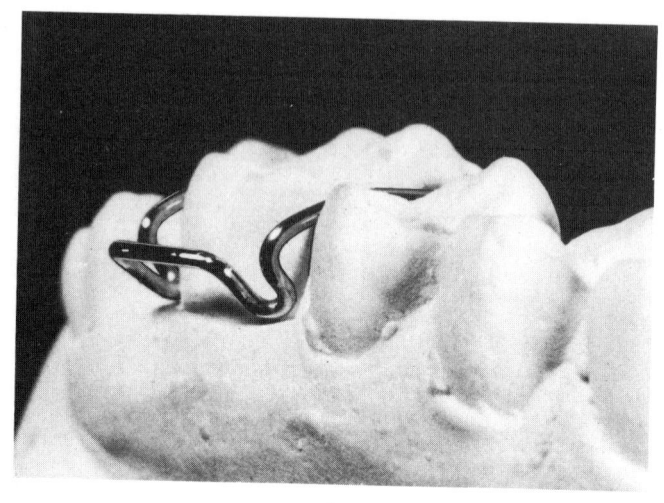

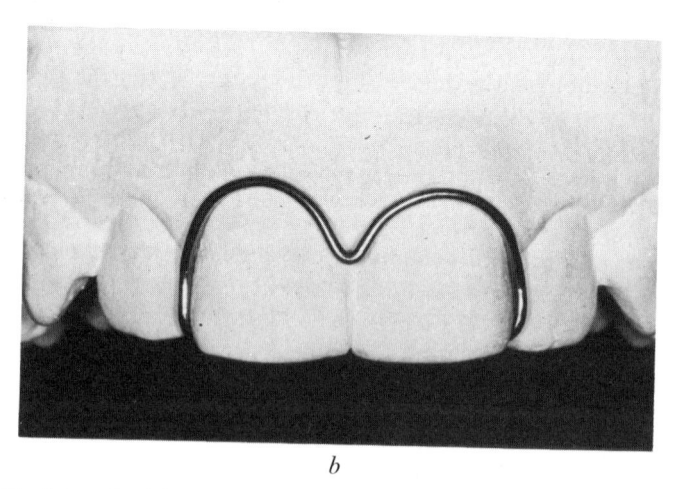

Fig. 8.4. *a*, An Adams' clasp. Note the arrowhead engages in undercuts on the mesiobuccal and distobuccal aspects of the molar but does not contact the adjacent teeth. *b*, A Southend clasp.

retention anteriorly. However, they are not very effective for this unless the incisors are proclined. It may be more efficient to use an Adams' clasp on the central incisors (*see Fig.* 9.6) but these should not be used on very proclined incisors because insertion of the appliance could be difficult. The Southend clasp (*see Fig.* 8.4b) is perhaps the most effective and unobtrusive form of anterior retention.

ANCHORAGE

Anchorage is provided by the sites which resist the forces of reaction generated by the active components of the appliance. The anchorage is thus the site from which the forces are applied.

The main sources of intra-oral anchorage are the teeth which are not to be moved and to which the appliance is attached by the retention components. The baseplate contacts the teeth and this also contributes to anchorage. In designing an appliance it is important to ensure that the anchorage is adequate. If it is not, the anchor teeth will be moved by the forces they are meant to resist and this will encroach on space required for the alignment of the irregular teeth. If the anchorage available within the one arch is considered to be insufficient, it should be reinforced (*see below*).

The resistance of a tooth to movement is related to:

1. The surface area of the roots.

2. The type of tooth movement permitted: teeth can be tipped more readily than they can be moved bodily. By designing the appliance so that the anchor teeth cannot tip, the anchorage is increased. However, although this is a common practice with fixed appliances, it is not easy with removable appliances.

3. Other factors such as the intercuspation of the teeth may contribute to the anchorage.

For descriptive purposes certain terms are used to

classify the various forms of anchorage:

Intramaxillary, where the teeth within the same arch are used as anchorage. This anchorage may be:

Simple where teeth of greater resistance are used as anchorage for movement of a tooth or teeth of lesser resistance.

Reciprocal where two teeth of equal resistance or two equal groups of teeth are used to move each other reciprocally to an equal extent in opposite directions.

Intermaxillary, where the other arch is used for anchorage. This anchorage may also be simple or reciprocal. Intermaxillary anchorage is most commonly used with fixed appliances where elastics are stretched from the front of one arch to the back of the other (the direction of pull depending on the case to be treated). However, this is rarely used with removable appliances because the elastics tend to displace the appliances and retention can be a problem. Certain functional appliances (e.g. the Andresen) use intermaxillary anchorage (*see* Chapter 18).

Extra-oral, where a headcap or neckstrap is used to provide or reinforce anchorage (*Fig.* 8.5). Extra-oral anchorage is a very useful adjunct to removable appliance therapy but appliances must be well made with good retention. The headcap has the advantage over a neckstrap in that traction can be directed in a slightly upward direction so that it does not tend to displace the appliance.

When extra-oral anchorage is used as reinforcement to intramaxillary anchorage, a removable facebow (*see Fig.* 9.2) or J hooks (*see Fig.* 9.3*b*) are used to transmit the forces to the appliance. The headgear should be worn at night and the force applied should be about twice that provided by the active component of the appliance.

Where anchorage is entirely extra-oral and the force is applied by extra-oral elastics, as in the 'En Masse' appliance for retraction of upper buccal segments (*see Fig.* 9.7), the appliance need be worn only with the headgear. For an acceptable rate of progress, the headgear and

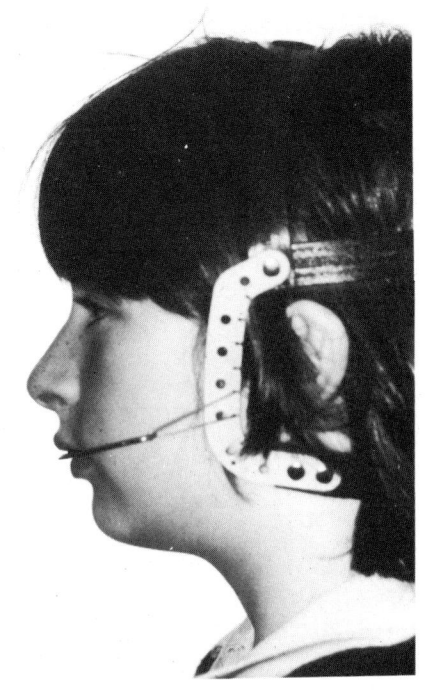

Fig. 8.5 Extra-oral anchorage with a headcap via a facebow.

appliance must be worn for more than 12 hours out of every 24. Many large-rooted teeth are being moved and so quite heavy forces are appropriate—up to 500 g (about 16 oz) in all.

It should be recognized that it is possible for J hooks or removable facebows to become disengaged, either during play or at night. A few cases have been reported where serious soft tissue laceration or even damage to an eye has resulted. Various types of safety headgear or safety straps are available to minimize the risk of this h•ppening, and these should be used routinely with J hooks or detachable facebows. Details of these are available from suppliers.

BASEPLATE

The framework of a removable appliance is an acrylic baseplate which: supports the wire components; contributes to anchorage by contacting the teeth which are not to be moved; prevents unwanted drift of teeth (although wire stops may be incorporated for this purpose (*see Fig.* 9.8)); transmits forces from the active components to the anchorage; protects palatal springs if they are boxed; and which may be extended to form anterior or posterior bite planes.

The baseplate should be as thin as possible to reduce bulk yet thick enough for strength. It should be closely adapted to all teeth except those which are to be moved.

Bite planes may be anterior or posterior. They are usually flat.

Anterior Bite Planes

These are used in order to reduce a deep overbite. They are also useful for relieving occlusal interference with tooth movement in cases where deepening of the overbite (which may occur if posterior planes are used) is to be avoided. Overbite reduction with an anterior bite plane depends largely on occlusal growth of the posterior teeth which are held out of occlusion. In the child this eruption of the posterior teeth would have occurred with facial growth and so the long term effect has been to prevent the lower labial segment from growing occlusally.

In Class II cases overbite reduction should be begun at the canine retraction stage. The bite plane should exceed the freeway space by 2–3 mm. The bite plane is also useful in removing occlusal interference to canine retraction. When the incisors are retracted a somewhat thicker plane should be constructed or a low plane may be thickened by additions of cold-cure acrylic. In trimming the bite plane to allow upper incisor retraction (*Fig.* 8.6) it is important

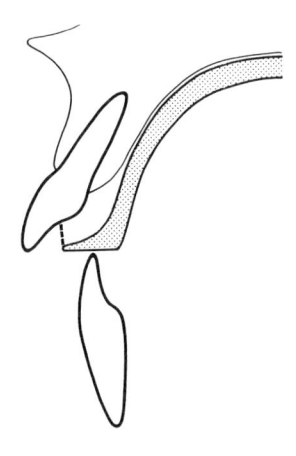

Fig. 8.6. Trimming an anterior bite plane to allow incisor retraction. So that the lower incisors will still occlude with it, the bite plane should not be trimmed back too far. Then it is undermined to clear it well away from the palatal surface of the upper incisors.

to clear it well away from these teeth yet to maintain contact with the lower incisors. It is useful when designing an appliance to record the size of overjet so that the technician can extend the bite plane by an appropriate amount.

Inclined anterior bite planes are sometimes used to reinforce anchorage through the distal components of biting forces. However, they are not very effective in this respect and may procline the lower incisors. For this reason they are not recommended.

Posterior Bite Planes

These are used to clear occlusal interferences to tooth movement (particularly where there is a mandibular displacement) in appliances for correction of unilateral crossbite (*see Fig.* 9.15) and instanding upper incisors (*see Fig.* 9.10). For comfort the occlusal coverage of the posterior teeth should be only just thick enough to clear the occlusion.

CONSTRUCTION AND REPAIR OF REMOVABLE APPLIANCES

Materials used

Stainless Steel

In orthodontic work 18 : 8 austenitic stainless steel wire is used: in hard form for springs, clasps and arch wires; and in soft form for ligatures and separating wires. It is stainless because the 18% chromium contributes resistance to oxidation by forming a passive surface film and the 8% nickel resists other forms of corrosion. The carbon content is kept as low as practical (less than 0·5%) as, on heating, chromium carbide tends to be deposited at grain boundaries, reducing corrosion resistance.

Advantages. Cheap, strong, resilient, not affected by the oral fluids, and fairly easy to manipulate.

Disadvantages. Must be worked in hard state but excessive working causes fatigue and fracture.

Soldering is difficult and requires special flux and even then union is poor. Special fluoride-containing fluxes are necessary to remove the passive surface film of chromium oxide. A low-fusing silver solder is most suitable.

The essential points to be observed are that the wires should be thoroughly cleaned, in close contact and liberally coated with flux. The area of the joint must be adequately heated using a gentle blue flame. The operation should be completed as rapidly as possible to minimize overheating and annealing the adjacent wire.

Welding. In orthodontic spot welding the pieces to be welded are held together under pressure and a current is passed. The resistance at the junction of the parts results in a rise in temperature and fusion occurs due to localized melting at the point of juncture. The grain structure of the wire should not be seriously affected. A high density low voltage current is used (100 A, 5 V) and the time of the weld is made very brief ($\frac{1}{100}$ sec) to avoid overheating of the wire adjacent to the weld.

Acrylic Resin

This is used for the baseplate. Removable orthodontic appliances are often heat-cured but there are advantages of speed and convenience in using cold-cure acrylic. Heat-cured acrylic is stronger. Clear acrylic is often preferred by the patient and has the advantage that it is possible to see blanching of the palatal mucosa in any areas where the baseplate needs to be relieved.

Construction. For details of the construction of removable appliances *see* Adams (1970). It has been emphasized that for successful use removable appliance components must be carefully made. The major points to look for in a palatal spring and in an Adams' clasp are illustrated in *Figs.* 8.2 and 8.4.

Repairs. Most fractures of appliances result from faults in design or construction, or abuse on the part of the patient. It is important that repairs can be done rapidly and conveniently. Some practitioners keep a duplicate of the model on which the appliance was made. Alternatively, an impression may be taken, preferably with the appliance in place.

Baseplate

Badly designed or badly fitting baseplates may fracture in use. However, most baseplate fractures occur when the appliance is out of the mouth. Self-curing acrylic is used for the repair.

Springs and Clasps

Occasionally these components can be readapted or repaired by soldering. However, this is rarely satisfactory and ideally the fractured component should be cut from the baseplate using a fissure burr, a new one bent up on the model and cured into the baseplate with cold-cure acrylic.

Chapter 9

Removable Appliances

The advantages and limitations of removable appliances compared with fixed appliances are described in Chapter 17. However, before considering orthodontic treatment it is important to be sure that the patient will benefit from treatment and is willing to wear appliances. A comprehensive treatment plan, in which the objectives of treatment are defined, must be formulated. Provided that these objectives can be achieved by simple tipping of the teeth, removable appliances will be satisfactory. Treatment planning for the various malocclusions is discussed in Chapters 12–16.

In this Chapter, a variety of removable appliances is described to illustrate the principles of removable appliance design. The appliance, with appropriate variations, should be designed by the dentist for each case. Instructions to the technician should include a careful drawing and a written description (*Fig.* 9.1). All wires (except for stops which are made in soft wire) are hard-drawn stainless steel and in the description diameters are given in millimetres.

APPLIANCE DESIGN

Appliances should be simple, comfortable, of minimal bulk and adequate strength. It is a mistake to try to undertake a large number of tooth movements with a single appliance. Appliance design will be considered under the following headings: (1) upper appliances for mesial or distal tooth movements; (2) upper appliances for labial (and buccal) or palatal tooth movements; (3) lower appliances; (4) passive appliances.

REMOVABLE APPLIANCES

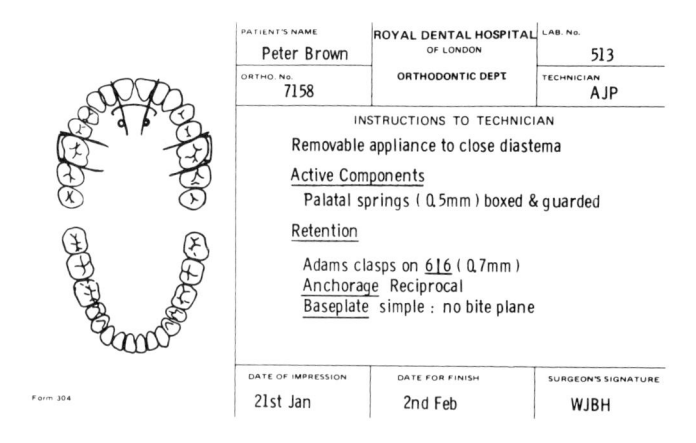

PATIENT'S NAME Peter Brown	ROYAL DENTAL HOSPITAL OF LONDON	LAB. No. 513
ORTHO. No. 7158	ORTHODONTIC DEPT	TECHNICIAN AJP
INSTRUCTIONS TO TECHNICIAN		
Removable appliance to close diastema		
Active Components Palatal springs (0.5mm) boxed & guarded		
Retention Adams clasps on 6│6 (0.7mm) Anchorage Reciprocal Baseplate simple : no bite plane		
DATE OF IMPRESSION 21st Jan	DATE FOR FINISH 2nd Feb	SURGEON'S SIGNATURE WJBH

Fig. 9.1. An appliance design should include a drawing and a careful description for the technician. This appliance will be used to approximate the central incisors.

UPPER APPLIANCES FOR MESIAL OR DISTAL TOOTH MOVEMENTS

Approximation of Upper Central Incisors (*Fig.* 9.1)

Active component. Palatal springs (0·5 mm) boxed and guarded.
Retention. Clasps on 6/6 (0·7 mm).
Anchorage. Reciprocal.
Baseplate. A simple baseplate unless there is occlusal interference with tooth movement in which case an anterior bite plane should be incorporated.
Point to note. See p. 118 for the indications for closure of a median diastema. A labial bow may be incorporated to prevent labial movement of the incisors during the mesial movement.

Retraction of Upper Canines

Basic Design
Where anchorage is not a problem (*Fig.* 9.2).

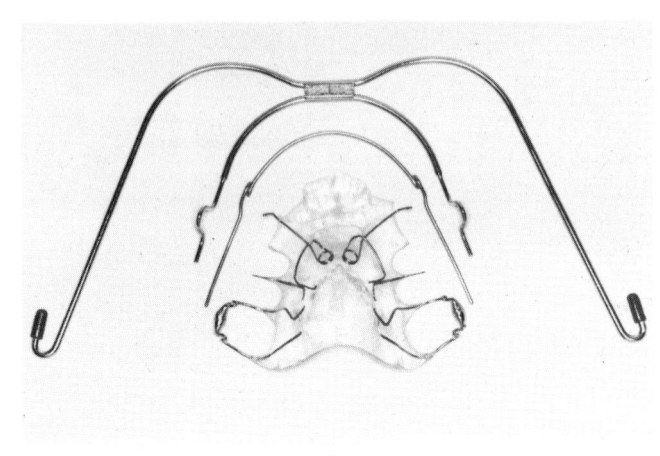

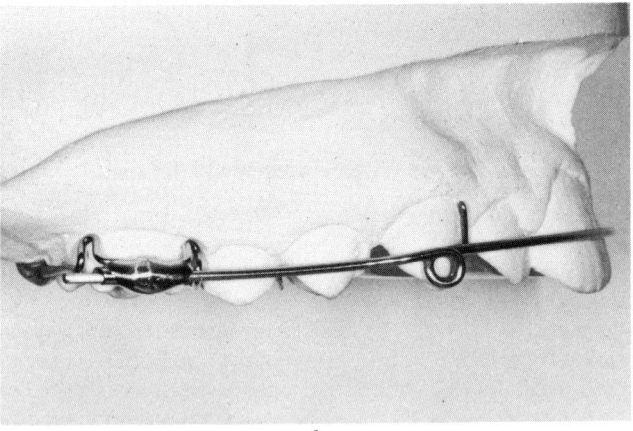

Fig. 9.2. *a,* A simple appliance to retract upper canines with palatal springs. It is usually wise to have tubes attached to the clasps on the molars so that, if required, a facebow (the outer bow) can be fitted to them and anchorage can be reinforced by extra-oral traction worn at nights. *b,* This simple appliance can be converted to retract the incisors in mild cases by the addition of a labial bow (shown detached in *a*). This bow slides into the tubes in the molar clasps and then light elastics can be placed over the ends of the tubes and the loops in the bow, to the incisors.

Active component. Palatal springs (0·5 mm) boxed and guarded. Buccally placed canines should be retracted using buccal springs (*Fig.* 9.3).

Retention. Adams clasps on 6|6 (0·7 mm)

Anchorage. Provided by teeth which are clasped and contacted by the baseplate.

Baseplate. An anterior bite plane is usually necessary to relieve occlusal interference and reduce the overbite if deep.

Points to note. The basic design without anchorage reinforcement is suitable only where the amount of retraction is quite small and anchorage is not at a premium. It may be found that the anchor teeth move forwards, encroaching on the space required for the canine retraction and producing an increase in overjet. Palatal springs should be activated in the free arm by about 3 mm; and buccal springs should be adjusted at the coil to give an activation of between 1 mm and 2 mm.

With Reinforced Anchorage

Where most of the space available is needed for canine retraction, anchorage must be reinforced. This is most effectively done by adding extra-oral anchorage to be worn at night (*see* p. 68).

Retention of the appliance must also be improved to resist displacement when the extra-oral anchorage is worn and a clasp on 1|1 is most effective. Some orthodontists use a fitted labial bow or cap the incisors to improve both anchorage and retention. However, their contribution to these functions is often not as great as may be desired.

With Provision for Reduction of a Small Overjet (less than 5 mm) or Alignment of Irregular Incisors (*Fig.* 9.4)

It is possible to incorporate a labial bow (in 0·7 mm wire) in the appliance which may later be used for incisor retraction or alignment. For details of incisor retraction *see* p. 82.

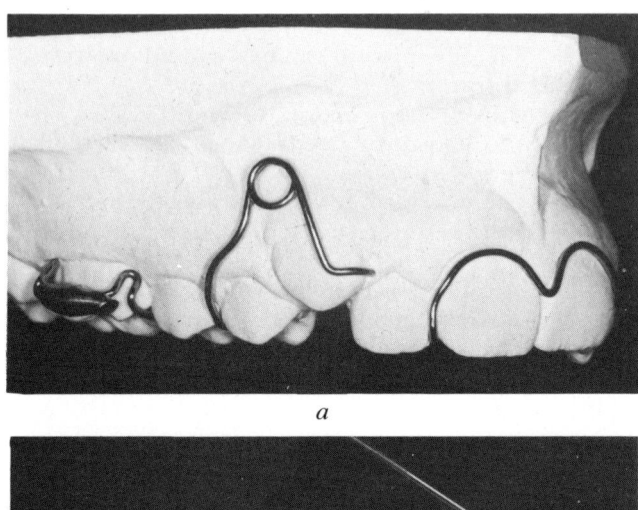

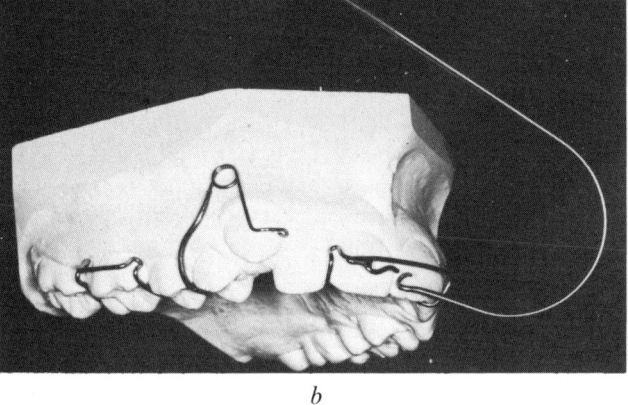

Fig. 9.3. *a*, Retraction of a buccally placed canine with a buccally placed spring in 0·7 mm wire. Tubes on the molar clasps provide for the use of extra-oral traction with a facebow if anchorage reinforcement is required. Self-supporting buccal springs like this are rather stiff and have a poor stability ratio which make adjustment difficult. *b*, A spring of 0·5 mm wire supported in tubing is more gentle than a self-supporting spring and is easier to adjust. This appliance illustrates spurs on an incisor clasp to which J hooks can be attached for anchorage reinforcement. As with a facebow (*Fig.* 8.5) the J hooks are attached to headgear by means of elastics.

REMOVABLE APPLIANCES 79

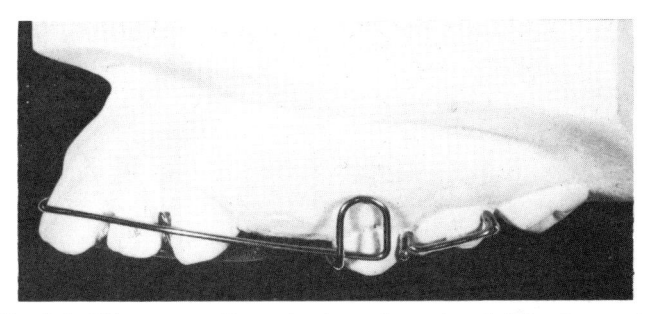

Fig. 9.4. Where a small overjet is to be reduced following canine retraction, it may be possible to do this with a labial bow incorporated in the same appliance. This will also prevent any buccal movement of the canines which can be produced by the palatal spring. The stability ratio of this bow is poor.

The labial bow is rather rigid and so this appliance should be used only in mild cases where the amount of tooth movement required is small. Other modifications to retract the incisors with the appliance which has been used to retract canines is the use of a latex elastic (*see Fig.* 8.3) or the addition of a sliding bow (*see Fig.* 9.2). For more severe cases it is better to retract the canines and incisors with separate appliances.

Retraction of Premolars following Loss of First Permanent Molars (*Fig.* 9.5)

Active component. Palatal springs on 5/5 and 4/4 (0·5 mm boxed and guarded).
Retention. Clasps on 7/7 and 3/3 (or 1/1). (0·7 mm.)
Anchorage. The teeth which are clasped and contacted by the baseplate. If space is at a premium, reinforce with extra-oral anchorage. J hooks to spurs on the canine clasps allow an upward and backward direction of traction which does not interfere with retention of the appliance.
Baseplate. If the overjet is to be reduced or if there is occlusal interference with the appliance or tooth

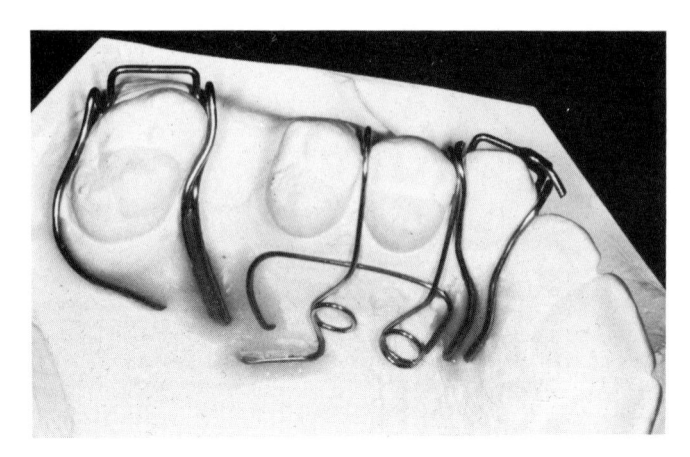

Fig. 9.5. The retraction of premolars following loss of first permanent molars.

movement, incorporate an anterior bite plane.
Points to note. The appliance should be fitted before or immediately after the extractions. Some operators fit a spur in contact with the mesial surface of the second molars (below the arm of the clasp). This means that the appliance has to be fitted after the extractions.

Palatal springs should be activated by about 3 mm.

Distal Movement of First Permanent Molars (*Fig.* 9.6)

Active component. Screws with the axis parallel to the line of the arch.
Retention. Clasps on 6|6 (0·7 mm) plus a clasp on 1/1 or a fitted labial bow. 4/4 should also be clasped if possible.
Anchorage. The teeth not being moved. Anchorage must be reinforced with extra-oral traction.
Baseplate. This should be split as indicated in the figure. An anterior bite plate may be used to clear the occlusion.

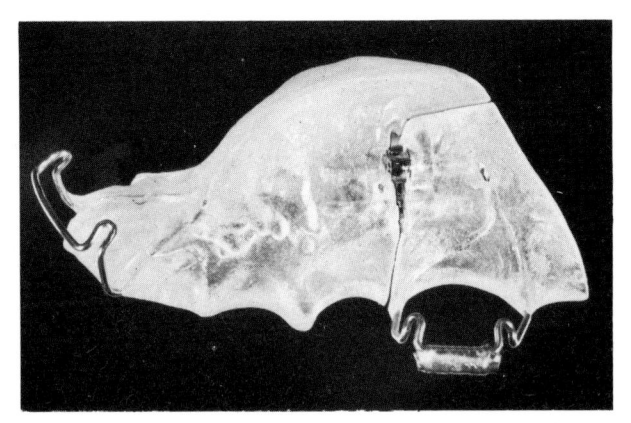

Fig. 9.6. Distal movement of upper first permanent molars with a screw plate. Anchorage is reinforced with extra-oral gear.

Point to note. This movement is difficult if 7/7 have erupted. It is better done, in cases where 6/6 have drifted forwards following early loss of deciduous molars, either before 7/7 have erupted or if they have been extracted.

Retraction of Upper Buccal Segments

The 'En Masse' appliance (*Fig.* 9.7).
Active component. The elastics of the headgear. A Coffin spring in 1·25 mm wire (or screw—*Fig.* 9.15) should be incorporated to allow the buccal segments to be expanded as they move distally. The arch diverges distally and slight expansion is required to preserve the correct transverse relationship with the lower arch. The patients should be seen at 6-week intervals when the appliance should be activated by the dentist as necessary.

The extra-oral forces are transmitted to the appliance through a face bow. The extra-oral part is 1·5 mm wire and the intra-oral part, which stands clear of the incisors,

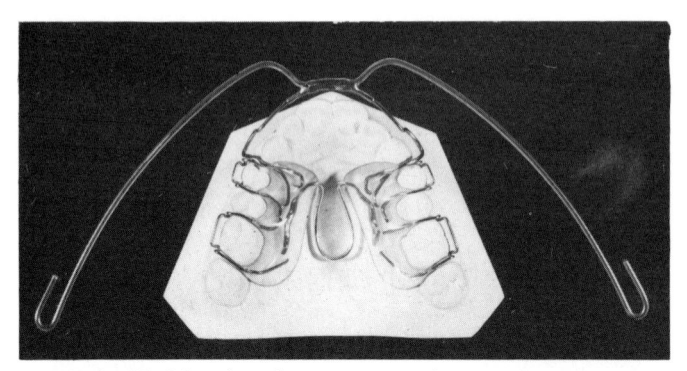

Fig. 9.7. An 'En Masse' appliance to retract the upper buccal segments.

is in 1·15 mm wire. The bow may be inserted directly into the baseplate or into tubes on molar clasps.
Retention. Clasps on 6/6 (0·7 mm) and 4/4 (0·6 mm).
Anchorage. Extra-oral.
Baseplate. Split in the midline and cut away from the upper incisors.
Points to note. To be effective the headgear must be worn for about 14 hours out of 24. Quite heavy forces—up to 250 g (about 8 oz) each side—are appropriate because many teeth have to be moved. The face bow should not contact the upper incisors and it may have to be adjusted at the loops to keep it clear as the buccal segments move distally.

UPPER APPLIANCES FOR LABIAL OR PALATAL TOOTH MOVEMENTS

Retraction of Upper Incisors

Roberts' Retractor (*Fig.* 9.8)
Active component. Retractor in 0·5 mm wire supported by tubing 0·5 mm internal diameter.
Retention. Clasps on 6/6 (0·7 mm).

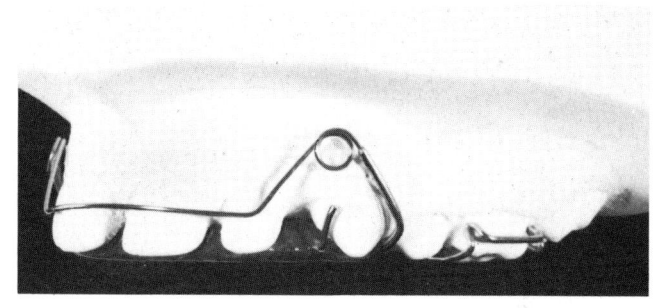

Fig. 9.8. A Roberts' retractor.

Anchorage. The teeth which are clasped and contacted by the baseplate.

Baseplate. Should incorporate stops mesial to 3|3 . There should be an anterior bite plane to reduce the overbite. In order to maintain control of the lower incisors while it is trimmed back clear of the upper incisors the bite plane should be at least two-thirds of the height of the upper incisors. It may be thickened by adding cold-cure acrylic.

Points to note. The Roberts' retractor should not be activated where it emerges from the tubes, otherwise it will fracture in use. The bite plane should be progressively trimmed back clear of the upper incisors as they are retracted, while still maintaining contact with the lower incisors (*see Fig.* 8.6). It is not possible to do this if the bite plane is too thin. Ideally, overbite reduction should have been completed at the canine retraction stage and the bite plane on this appliance maintains the reduction. However, in some cases further overbite reduction is needed.

Labial Bows (*Fig.* 9.9)

These are made from 0·7 mm wire and so are less flexible but more robust than the Roberts' retractor. Various designs of labial bow are used but it is important that the amount of wire in the loop is as large as possible to increase flexibility.

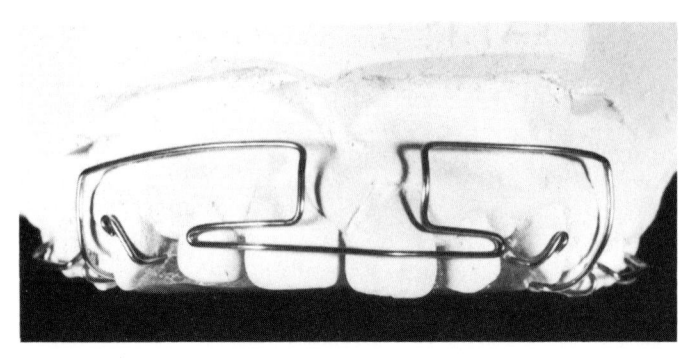

Fig. 9.9. A Mills' bow to retract the upper incisors.

The appliance illustrated in *Fig.* 9.4 (p. 79) can be modified to retract the upper incisors by carefully activating the labial bow. If an overjet is to be reduced, the bow should be activated by opening up the reverse loops. These labial bows are quite rigid and the amount of activation must be small (about 1 mm).

Proclination of Upper Incisors (*Fig.* 9.10)

Active component. Boxed finger springs or Z springs, the number and diposition depending on the number of instanding teeth.

Retention. Clasps on 6/6 (0·7 mm) and, as the springs tend to displace the plate downwards, on 4/4 or D/D (0·6 mm).

Anchorage. The teeth which are clasped. Anchorage is not usually a problem.

Baseplate. This protects the springs. In general, if incisor proclination is to be stable there will be an overbite and so it is advantageous to clear the occlusion by capping the posterior teeth to give a thin posterior bite plane.

Points to note. It is usually important to avoid depressing the upper incisors and so T springs (*see Fig.* 9.14*a*), which are very convenient for buccal movement of premolars,

REMOVABLE APPLIANCES 85

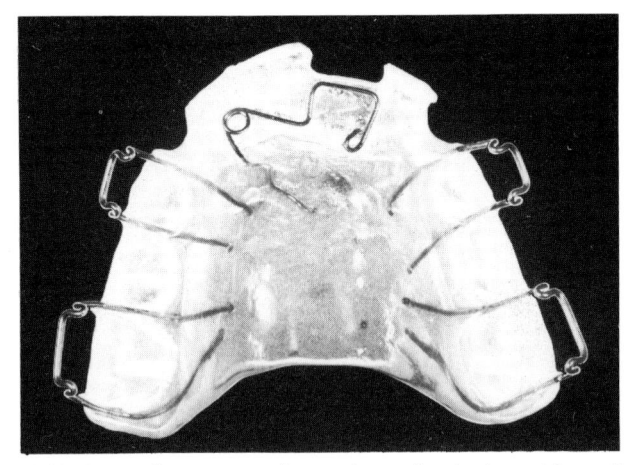

Fig. 9.10. An appliance to procline an instanding incisor with a palatal finger spring. Note that it is cranked to avoid contact with the other incisors.

but have a large intrusive component and limited range, are best avoided. Individual spring-loaded screws may be used but they are expensive. Where the four upper incisors are instanding, a screw plate (*Fig.* 9.11) may be

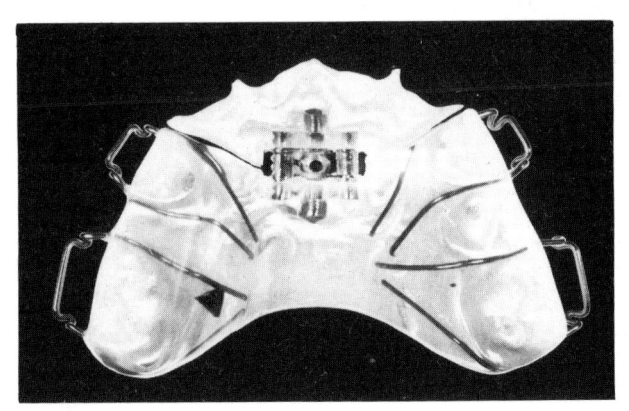

Fig. 9.11. A screw plate to procline four upper incisors.

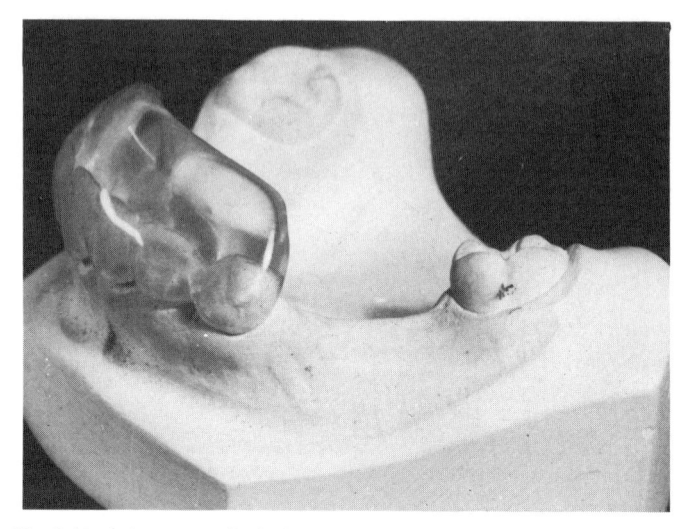

Fig. 9.12. A lower acrylic inclined plane to be cemented onto the lower incisors. This can be used to procline instanding upper incisors.

used. This is activated by the patient but does make the appliance rather bulky.

Where upper first molar teeth are missing and retention of the appliance would be a problem a lower inclined plane may be used. This may be incorporated into a removable appliance or cemented as a splint to the lower incisors (*Fig.* 9.12). If such an appliance has not proved effective within 1 month it should be abandoned because it is rather traumatic. More conventional treatment can be carried out when more teeth have erupted.

Palatal Movement of Canines and Premolars

Active component. A self-supporting buccal spring (0·7 mm) (*Fig.* 9.13).
Retention. Clasps on 6/6 and if necessary on 1/1 (0·7 mm).

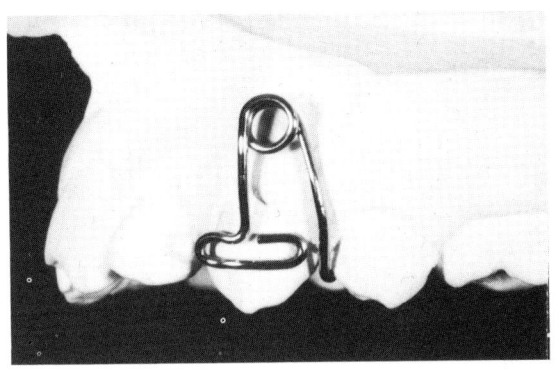

Fig. 9.13. A buccal spring to move a canine palatally. A similar design may be used for palatal movement of premolar teeth.

Anchorage. The other teeth which are contacted by the baseplate.
Baseplate. A bite plane should be incorporated if there would be occlusal interference to the tooth movement. In order not to affect adversely the overbite the bite plane should be anterior if the overbite is deep, posterior if the overbite is small.

Buccal Movement of Canines and Premolars (*Fig.* 9.14*a* and *b*)

Active component. T springs (0·5 mm) (*Fig.* 9.14*a*) are preferred to Z springs in the premolar area because they are simpler for the patient to insert. In the canine area it may be better to use a cranked finger spring (*Fig.* 9.14*b*) to avoid intruding the tooth.
Retention. Clasps on 6|6 and if possible on the central incisors or at least one first premolar (0·7 mm).
Anchorage. The other teeth which are contacted by the baseplate.
Baseplate. Molar capping may be necessary to clear occlusal interference to the tooth movement.

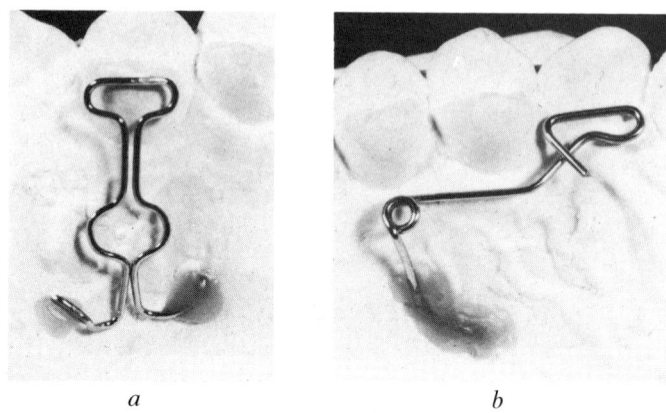

Fig. 9.14. *a*, A T spring to move a premolar buccally. It is adjusted by pulling it away from the baseplate. It may be lengthened at the adjustment loops as the tooth moves. *b*, A cranked finger spring to move a canine buccally.

Upper Arch Expansion (*Fig.* 9.15)

Active component. Screw (or Coffin spring, 1·25 mm).
Retention. Clasps on 6/6 and 4/4.
Anchorage. The expansion should be symmetrical and so the anchorage is reciprocal.

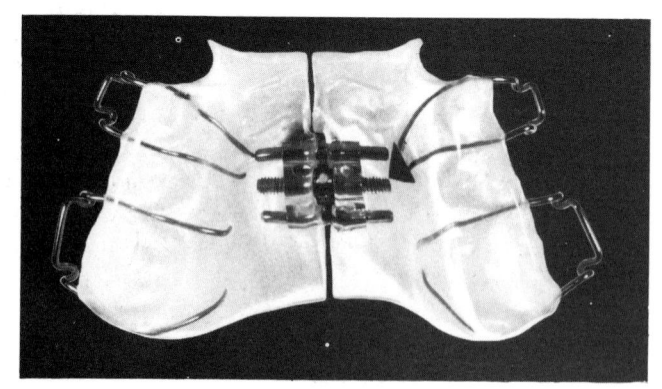

Fig. 9.15. An appliance to expand the upper arch.

Baseplate. Cut away from the upper incisors and split in the midline. The baseplate should be carried over the occlusal surfaces of the cheek teeth as thin capping to eliminate occlusal interferences.

Points to note. Expansion of this type should be undertaken only where there is a unilateral crossbite with lateral displacement (*see* p. 133). The screw should be activated by the patient by a quarter turn once or twice each week.

LOWER REMOVABLE APPLIANCES

Lower removable appliances are comparatively little used because:

1. The form of the lower arch is usually accepted and so buccolingual tooth movements are rarely indicated. In crowded cases, spontaneous alignment usually follows well-chosen extractions. This will not occur where the tooth inclinations are unfavourable but a fixed appliance would be required in these cases.

2. Lower removable appliances encroach on tongue space and, because the undercuts utilized by clasps may not be present in children, retention may be poor. However, well-made lower removable appliances may be used in selected cases. Only two examples are given.

It is important that the technician blocks out any undercuts on the lingual side of the alveolar process before the appliance is made, otherwise extensive trimming will be required, which is time consuming and which will weaken the appliance. If they are carelessly handled, lower removable appliances will fracture in the midline. The acrylic must be thick enough to provide reasonable strength without being unduly bulky.

Retraction of Lower Canines (*Fig.* 9.16)

Active component. Self-supporting buccal springs (0·7 mm) or supported springs in 0·5 mm wire.

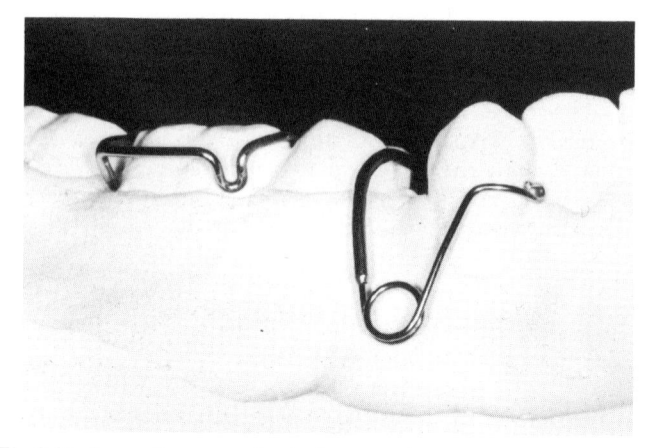

Fig. 9.16. An appliance to retract a lower canine.

Retention. Clasps on $\overline{6/6}$ (0·7 mm) possibly supplemented by a fitted labial bow on the lower incisors.
Anchorage. The other teeth and alveolar process.
Baseplate. Must be thick enough lingual to $\overline{3/3}$ to allow for trimming. Particulary if there is occlusal interference to the tooth movement, thin molar capping may be incorporated.

Distal Movement of Lower First Molars (*Fig.* 9.17)

This may be indicated where these teeth have drifted forwards following early loss of $\overline{E/E}$ and where extraction of premolars is not indicated. The movement is more readily achieved before $\overline{7/7}$ have erupted or if they have been extracted.
Active component. Narrow screws.
Retention. Clasps on $\overline{4/4}$ (0·6 mm) and $\overline{6/6}$ and fitted labial bow (0·7 mm).

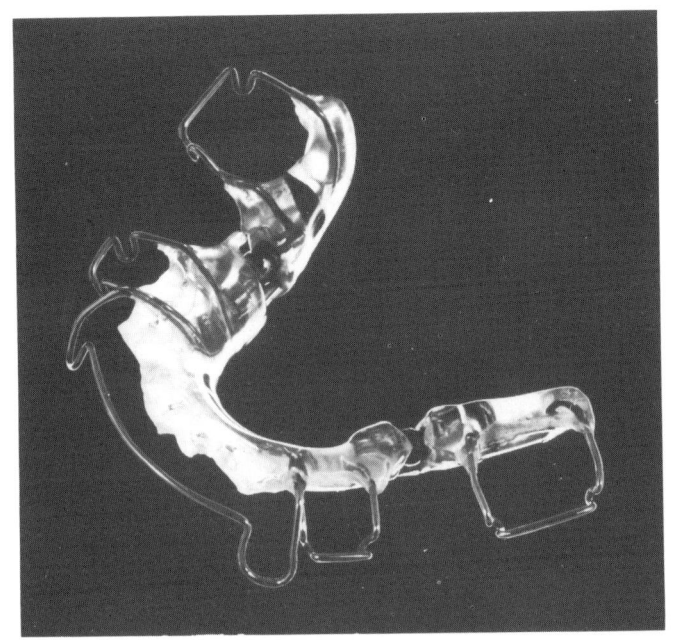

Fig. 9.17. Distal movement of lower molars with a screw plate.

Anchorage. The teeth not being moved and the alveolar process which is contacted by the baseplate.
Baseplate. Split at screws.
Points to note. Anchorage may be a problem and it is difficult to avoid proclining the lower incisors. Each screw should be activated once a week but on different days.

PASSIVE APPLIANCES

Space maintainers. These may be fitted following early loss of deciduous teeth (*but see* p. 99). Where premolars are extracted before permanent canines have fully erupted and no active tooth movement is required, a space maintainer may be indicated to preserve space until the canines have erupted fully.

Retainers. In most circumstances the last active appliance is made passive and used as a retainer. Where the active component is very flexible, as in the case of the Roberts' retractor, a more rigid retainer may be required. Such an appliance can usually be modified by taking an impression, bending up a labial bow in 0·7mm wire, removing the old active component and processing in the new one with cold-cure acrylic. However, particularly following fixed appliance treatment, a new retention appliance may be made. The most commonly used design is illustrated in *Fig.* 9.18.

INSTRUCTIONS TO PATIENTS

Clear instruction must be given when the appliance is fitted. Too many instructions are confusing.

1. Appliances should be worn at all times, including meals. The only exceptions are contact sports when the appliance should be left out.

2. The appliance should be removed and cleaned, and the teeth cleaned, if possible, after every meal.

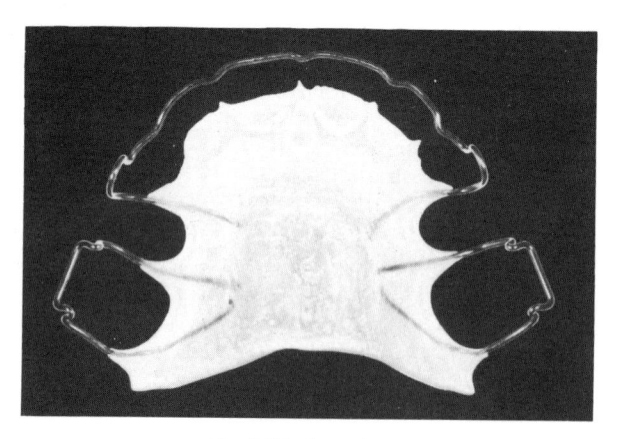

Fig. 9.18. A retainer.

3. The patient should be warned that it will take 1 or 2 days to get used to the appliance and that perseverence is important. If the appliance is damaged or cannot be worn for any reason, the dentist must be informed.

4. If headgear is worn to reinforce anchorage, it should be worn for at least 8 hours each night. Headgear used to retract buccal segments should be worn for at least 12 hours (preferably more) out of every 24.

ADJUSTMENT OF APPLIANCES

The patient should be seen every 4–6 weeks. At these visits, after asking the patient whether there have been any problems, the following routine should be adopted.

1. Check the general condition of the mouth: plaque, caries, gingival inflammation, soft tissue damage by the appliance.
2. Check for tooth movement:
a. Of the anchorage teeth: if the anchorage teeth have moved, either reduce the forces or reinforce anchorage.
b. Of the teeth that it is intended to move: a rate 1 mm per month is reasonable. Lack of tooth movement is usually due to interference from the baseplate or occlusion, incorrect activation, or failure of the patient to wear the appliance.
c. Record in the notes the changes in the occlusion.
3. If the tooth movement has not been completed:
a. Check that the teeth are still free to move.
b. Adjust the active component (if this is necessary).
c. Ensure that the patient can still insert the appliance.

Chapter 10

Local Factors in the Aetiology of Malocclusion

It is convenient to discuss local factors under the following headings: anomalies in the number of teeth; anomalies in the form and developmental position of teeth; habits and other local factors.

ANOMALIES IN THE NUMBER OF TEETH

1. Developmentally missing teeth.
2. Early loss of deciduous teeth.
3. Loss of permanent teeth.
4. Retained deciduous teeth.
5. Supernumerary teeth.

Developmentally Missing Teeth

Anodontia

The total failure of development of all teeth is a rare condition due to aplasia of the dental lamina. It is often associated with ectodermal dysplasia, an hereditary condition in which there is dry coarse skin, sparse hair, defects of the nails and absence of sweat glands. Anodontia is a prosthetic problem but it should be noted that the growth of the facial skeleton (apart from the alveolar processes of maxilla and mandible which are absent) is usually within normal limits.

Hypodontia

The developmental absence of a number of teeth is sometimes associated with ectodermal dysplasia as in the case of anodontia. In these cases, the teeth that are present are often conical in form and reduced in size. These patients present a major dental problem and partial dentures or bridges are required. Where possible, treatment of this sort should be delayed until the patient is old enough to maintain an excellent standard of oral hygiene while wearing a prosthesis.

Far more common than either of the conditions described above is the absence of a few teeth in an otherwise perfectly normal child. The teeth most commonly missing are third molars, upper lateral incisors, lower second premolars and upper second premolars.

Third molars. The absence of these teeth is not an orthodontic problem. However, if it is not intended to extract second permanent molars as part of orthodontic treatment, the presence of third molars of adequate size and in favourable positions must be confirmed. It should be remembered that the time of formation of third molars is very variable: frequently they are visible on radiographs at 8 years of age but occasionally they may not start to develop until 14 years.

Upper lateral incisors. The absence of these teeth presents an aesthetic problem. Sometimes in a crowded arch the canine will erupt in approximal contact with the central incisor and it may be reasonable to accept this position, merely reshaping the canine and building it up with composite as appropriate. More commonly, the canine will erupt close to but not in contact with the central incisor. A decision has to be made whether to close the space (which is functionally preferable) or whether to open it up for a prosthetic replacement for the lateral incisor (which may be aesthetically superior).

Closure of the space is indicated where there is crowding in the arch, where the canine is distally inclined or vertical so that it can readily be moved mesially, and where the appearance of the canine is acceptable to the patient. If the canine is mesially inclined a fixed appliance will be required to move the apex mesially as well. It may then be necessary to move the premolars mesially to close the space from behind.

Space opening is indicated where the canine is of a poor form so that the appearance would not be acceptable to the patient or where there is generalized spacing. If the arch is crowded, extractions will be required to provide space for retraction of the canine; and unless the canine is mesially inclined a fixed appliance will be required to retract it.

In summary, it is preferable to close the space of the lateral incisor in order to avoid the necessity for a prosthesis, provided that the appearance will be acceptable to the patient.

Second premolars. It is important that the absence of second premolars should be recognized as early as possible. However, the time of calcification is variable and in a few cases they may not become visible on radiographs until 7 years of age. It is essential always to check that second premolars are present before other teeth are extracted for orthodontic reasons.

Where there is crowding or an overjet has to be reduced, the space provided by the absence of the second premolars should be utilized. Where there is no crowding it is usually best to try to retain the second deciduous molars for as long as possible: they may be retained until the patient is 30 or 40 years of age. When they are shed the space will not normally close and, unless there are unopposed teeth in the other arch, little occlusal change may follow. Ideally a bridge should be fitted.

In some cases where a second premolar is missing the second deciduous molar may submerge (*see Fig.* 10.7). In the growing patient with a developing occlusion this may lead to quite severe drifting of the first permanent molar. The most satisfactory treatment in these cases is to close the gap using a fixed appliance to bring forward the permanent molar following removal of the submerged molar.

Early Loss of Deciduous Teeth

The effects of early loss depend on a number of factors including: (*a*) The tooth lost, (*b*) The age of loss, (*c*) Crowding.

The Tooth Lost

Deciduous incisors. Except in very crowded cases, early loss of carious deciduous incisors has little effect on the development of the occlusion. Where crowding is severe, space closure may occur but space maintenance is not indicated in the caries-prone mouth. If a deciduous incisor is intruded by a blow, displacement or dilaceration of the successor may result (*see* p. 114).

Deciduous canines. The early loss of these teeth is followed by a space loss as a result of alignment of crowded permanent incisors. The buccal segments may drift forwards by a small amount. Early loss of a deciduous canine, particularly in the lower arch, may result from resorption of its root by a crowded permanent lateral incisor. This is often unilateral and so the crowded incisors will drift to the side of loss with a shift of midline. This is the most serious result of early loss of a deciduous canine because it produces an asymmetrical occlusion which can be difficult to treat unless the midline is corrected. In order to avoid these complications it is good practice to balance the early loss of one deciduous canine by extracting the other deciduous canine from that arch.

Deciduous molars. Loss of contact areas due to caries may produce effects similar to early loss of deciduous teeth. The major effect of early loss of a second deciduous molar is that it allows forward movement of the first permanent molar, which encroaches on space for the premolars (*Fig.* 10.1). Space loss is usually more severe in the upper arch.

Early loss of a first deciduous molar also results in loss of space for the premolars, partly through forward drift of the posterior teeth as in the case of the second deciduous molar and partly as a result of relief of incisor crowding as in the case of the deciduous canine. The space loss from

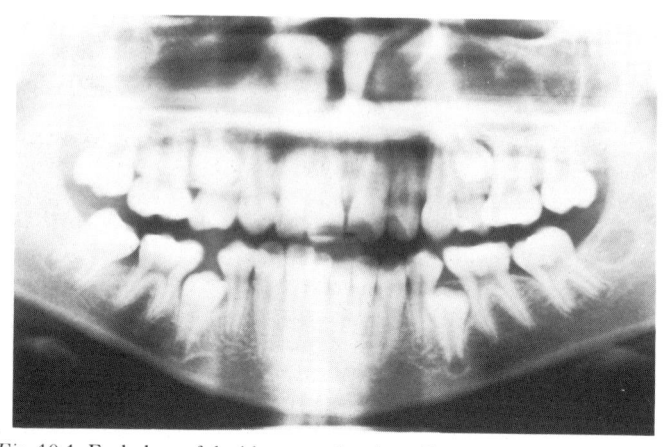

Fig. 10.1. Early loss of deciduous molars has allowed the first permanent molars to drift forwards, encroaching on the space for the second premolars.

forward drift of the buccal segment is not usually marked, but if the loss is unilateral the centre line will shift to that side. For this reason, as with deciduous canines, it is wise to balance the loss of one first deciduous molar by the extraction of the other from that arch at the same time. This is usually preferable to fitting a space maintainer for the reasons discussed below (p. 99).

Age of Loss

In general, the earlier the deciduous tooth is lost the more severe space loss will be.

Crowding

This is of major importance in determining the effects of early loss of deciduous teeth If the arch is spaced the effects of early loss are minor, whereas if there is crowding space loss may be severe.

Treatment
Where possible, carious deciduous molars, second molars in particular, should be adequately restored. However, where one first deciduous molar or a deciduous canine is lost, the simplest treatment is to balance this by extraction of the corresponding tooth on the opposite side of that arch. This will prevent a shift of midline which is often one of the greatest long term problems following early loss of such a tooth. Balancing extraction for the loss of a second deciduous molar is not usually indicated, but where a second deciduous molar is lost from an otherwise good mouth a space maintainer should be considered.

Space maintainers. May be removable or fixed (*Fig.* 10.2).

There are a number of problems associated with the use of space maintainers, including the danger of increased food stagnation and lack of patient cooperation, and so they should be fitted only in selected cases where they will be of positive benefit to the patient. Their use should be confined to the good, dentally aware patient who has lost one or perhaps two deciduous molars and where it is felt that orthodontic treatment might be avoided or considerably simplified by the prevention of space loss. Thus space maintainers are not indicated for the patient with spacing (where space loss will not occur anyway), or with moderate crowding (when extraction of permanent teeth and orthodontic treatment will be needed). Where it is estimated that there is just sufficient room for all the permanent teeth or, in the severely crowded case, where the extraction of one permanent tooth from each quadrant will provide just enough space, space maintainers may offer definite advantages.

Loss of Permanent Teeth

The permanent teeth most commonly extracted because of caries are first molars while upper incisors may be lost due to trauma. Both situations present major orthodontic problems.

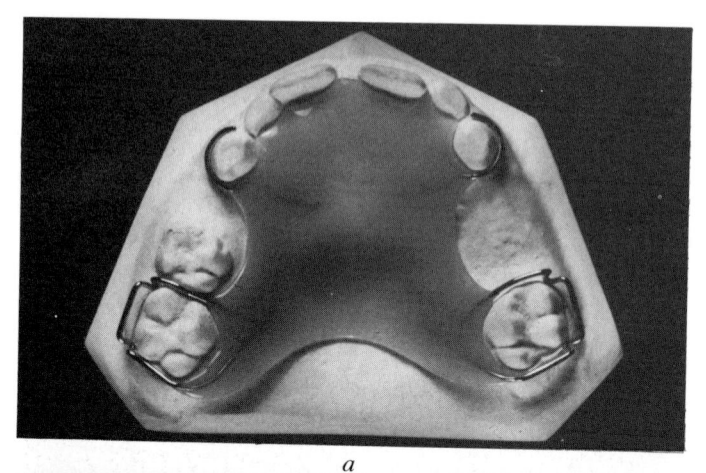

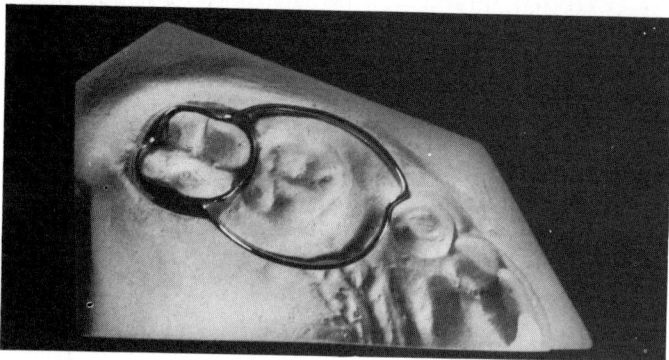

Fig. 10.2. *a*, A removable space maintainer. *b*, A simple fixed space maintainer.

Upper Incisors

Loss of these teeth is more common where they are prominent as in a Class II division 1 incisor relationship. Following such an accident, the first concern must be for the general wellbeing of the patient and then attempts may be made to save the tooth (if there has been a fracture) or to reimplant it (if it has been avulsed). Should these measures fail, an orthodontic treatment plan has to be formulated. The basic choice lies between utilization of the space (to relieve crowding or reduce an overjet) or maintenance of the space for a prosthesis. A positive policy must be followed and teeth adjacent to the gap should not be allowed to drift in an uncontrolled fashion. This would produce an unsightly, partially closed space which is difficult to deal with. Thus unless controlled space closure with an orthodontic appliance is to be undertaken, a single-tooth denture should be fitted as a space maintainer (*Fig.* 10.3). (It may be mentioned that

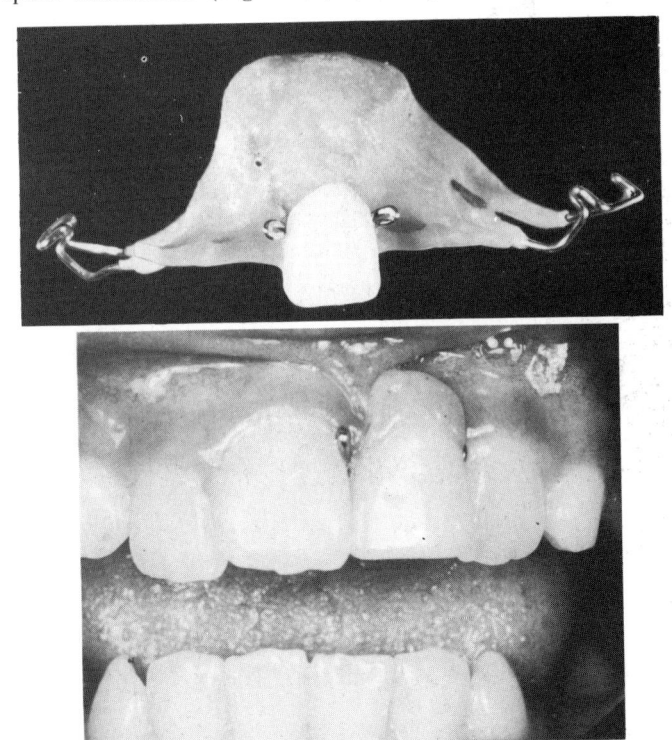

Fig. 10.3. A single-tooth denture as a space maintainer. Note the spurs in contact with the teeth on either side of the gap. These ensure that there will be no space loss.

where an upper incisor has been fractured, contact areas should be restored as soon as possible to prevent uncontrolled drift.)

Usually the best aesthetic result is obtained by fitting a prosthesis to replace the missing incisor and treating the coexisting malocclusion on its merits. This may involve extraction of other teeth. Sometimes the space of the missing incisor may be used to relieve crowding or reduce an overjet. To obtain an acceptable appearance it is then usually necessary to crown the lateral incisor on the side of loss to simulate a central incisor. This is not a simple solution to the problem because it is often necessary to move bodily the incisors adjacent to the space, with a fixed appliance; and it is not easy to make a good crown if the lateral incisor is small. However, in suitable cases it may be worth closing the space as described to avoid the need for a denture or bridge.

First Permanent Molars

These are never the teeth of choice for orthodontic extraction. However, if their condition is poor they may have to be removed and the space utilized for orthodontic treatment. The timing of extraction is very important: if they are removed in the mixed dentition period the effects are much less harmful than if they are extracted later. It is therefore essential to assess the life expectancy of a first molar that requires extensive restoration as early as possible and if the prognosis is poor, serious consideration should be given to its extraction at that time rather than leaving it to be extracted later. It is also important that, before first molars are extracted, an orthodontic treatment plan is formulated. It is often possible to minimize the harmful effects of first molar extractions and to avoid the need for later orthodontic treatment by balancing extractions at the optimal time.

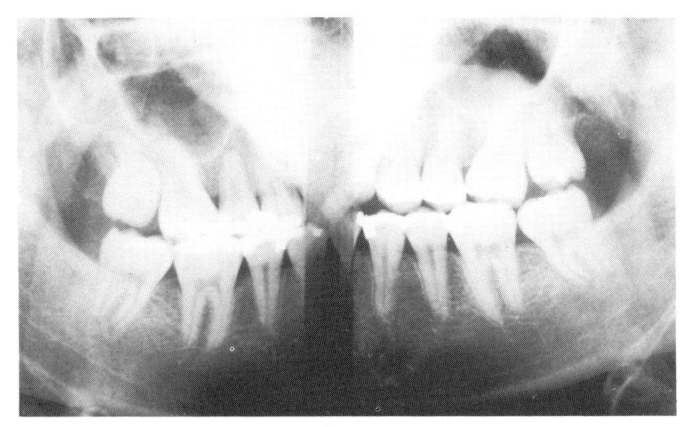

Fig. 10.4. The first permanent molars were extracted at the optimal time, just as root formation of the second permanent molars was beginning. The second molars have established a good contact relationship with the second premolars and space has been provided for eruption of the third molars.

Extraction in the mixed dentition

THE LOWER ARCH—if a first permanent molar is extracted before the eruption of the second premolar and second permanent molar, space closure will occur partly as a result of the forward eruption of the second molar and partly through distal drift of the second premolar (*Fig.* 10.4). This will relieve crowding in the premolar and canine region and mild or moderate incisor crowding will also improve. If the extraction is unilateral the centre line will drift to that side producing an asymmetric malocclusion. The contact between the second premolar and second permanent molar is rarely ideal, because the teeth tip towards one another, but it is usually reasonable. Sometimes the lower second premolar will drift distally to a marked extent, leaving a space distal to the first premolar (*Fig.* 10.5). While this is not an ideal occlusal arrangement, it is usually functionally acceptable and the space is large enough to avoid food packing.

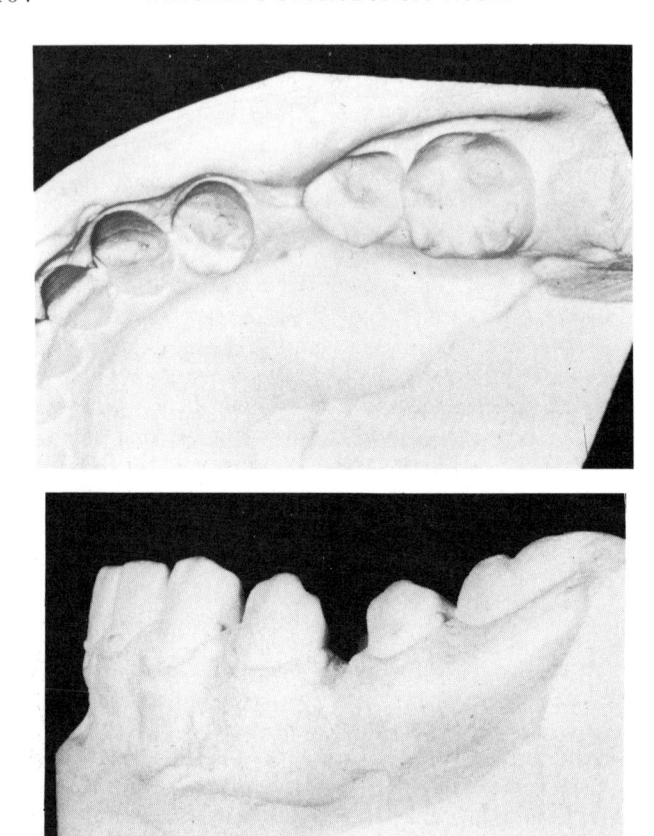

Fig. 10.5. The second premolar has drifted distally following early loss of the first permanent molar.

THE UPPER ARCH—the major part of the extraction space is closed through forward drift of the second permanent molar. If the premolars are crowded due to previous forward drift of the first permanent molar, following early loss of a deciduous molar, this will be relieved. A certain amount of improvement in incisor crowding may follow but this is variable and is less than in the lower arch.

Frequently, the second permanent molar will be slightly mesiopalatally rotated but the contact relationship with the second premolar is fair.

Extraction in the permanent dentition
THE LOWER ARCH—the effects of extractions of the first permanent molar after the second permanent molar has erupted are often disastrous: the second molar will tip forward and roll lingually; a very poor contact may be established with the second premolar (*Fig.* 10.6) but usually a stagnation area is produced; secondary changes in the upper arch often follow producing occlusal disharmonies and plunger cusp mechanisms. There will be little spontaneous improvement in incisor crowding. These effects are particularly marked where the extraction has been performed while the patient is still growing. In the adult, drift of the second molar is less marked and the result is often less harmful although unopposed upper teeth may over erupt.

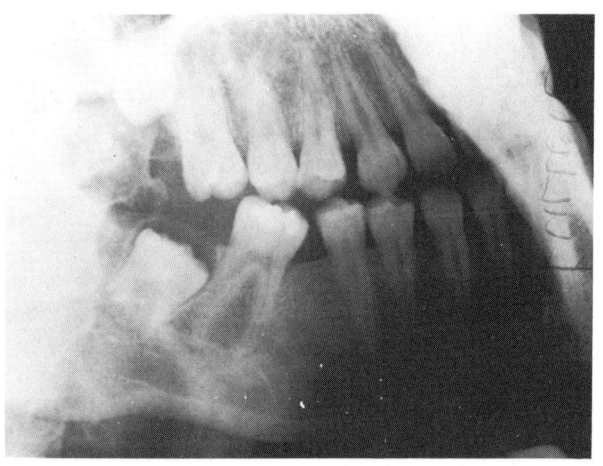

Fig. 10.6. The first permanent molars were extracted after the second permanent molars had erupted. Particularly in the lower arch the result is poor.

THE UPPER ARCH—space closure is better than in the lower arch and it occurs largely through mesial tipping and mesiopalatal rotation of the upper second molar around its palatal root.

Treatment planning in the mixed dentition for the patient who must lose first permanent molars. It is emphasized that the rules for balancing extraction of first permanent molars discussed below apply only in the mixed dentition and where there is no spacing. In the permanent dentition balancing extraction should not be performed unless the space is required for appliance treatment; in the mixed dentition balancing extraction should be carried out particularly where subsequent appliance treatment is contraindicated.

The following discussion is based upon the condition that all other permanent teeth (except perhaps third molars) are present, sound and in favourable positions. If this is not so, the treatment plan will have to be modified accordingly.

The best time for extraction of the first permanent molar is just after root formation of the second permanent molar has begun. This is usually between the ages of $8\frac{1}{2}$ and $10\frac{1}{2}$ years. The timing is more critical in the lower than in the upper arch.

CLASS I MALOCCLUSIONS—in the lower arch if one first permanent molar is in poor condition both should be removed at the optimal time. This will allow maximal relief of crowding and a fair contact relationship between the second premolar and the second permanent molar. The balancing extraction of the other first molar preserves the symmetry of the arch, relieves crowding on the other side and removes a tooth which may well also be cariously involved. If the upper arch is mildly crowded and particularly where there has been forward drift of the permanent molars, extraction of both upper first permanent molars at the same time as the lowers is indicated. However, if the upper arch is very crowded and if the upper first permanent molars are sound, it is preferable not to extract them but at a later stage to remove teeth nearer the site of crowding (for example, first premolars).

If one upper first permanent molar has to be extracted, the other should be removed at the same time to preserve symmetry but compensating extractions should not be undertaken in the lower arch. Should the upper arch crowding not resolve spontaneously, retraction of the upper buccal segments using extra-oral traction will be necessary.

Sometimes it is suggested that in crowded cases the first permanent molars should be retained until the second permanent molars erupt and can be held back while appliances are used to retract teeth anterior to the extraction space. In the lower arch a fixed appliance is required; in the upper a removable appliance may be used but treatment is prolonged and the results are often poor.

Occasionally, if crowding is very severe, it is necessary to extract two teeth from each quadrant. In these cases the first permanent molars should be extracted early following the guidelines indicated above and then, when the permanent canines have emerged into the mouth, the first premolars are extracted. It must be emphasized that these cases requiring the removal of two teeth from each quadrant are rare, and if there is any doubt premolars should not be extracted but the residual crowding accepted.

CLASS II MALOCCLUSIONS—as far as the extraction of first permanent molars is concerned, the two divisions of Class II can be considered together. If a lower first permanent molar is grossly carious at an early age, both lower first molars should be extracted at the optimal time but compensating extractions of first molars from the upper arch are not indicated unless they have a poor prognosis. The upper arch can then be treated on its merits, usually with extraction of first premolars at the appropriate time.

If the upper first permanent molars are of doubtful prognosis, it is usually best to extract them early and then treat the upper arch on its merits: the occlusion may be accepted or, where space requirements are slight, the upper buccal segments may be retracted using headgear; but if considerable space is necessary, upper first premolars may be removed and the overjet reduced.

As in crowded Class I cases, the practice of patching up first permanent molars until second molars have erupted and then moving back premolars into the extraction space, commits the patient to a long and unsatisfactory treatment procedure. This may be unavoidable where the poor prognosis of the first molars is not apparent until the early permanent dentition. However, if first permanent molars are removed early, spontaneous improvement of crowding (but not of overjet) will take place, and should the patient prove to be unsuitable for orthodontic treatment they can be left as they are. If treatment is indicated the retraction of the buccal segments with extra-oral anchorage (p. 143) is simpler and gives a better result than the individual tipping of premolars.

CLASS III MALOCCLUSIONS—In general, if one first permanent molar is carious it should be extracted early and, provided that the arch is crowded, a balancing extraction of the first molar from the opposite side should be undertaken. Thus if one lower first permanent molar is of poor life expectancy, both lower first molars should be extracted and the upper arch treated on its merits. Equally if one upper first permanent molar has to be extracted early, the other should be removed at the same time and lower arch treatment planned as discussed in Chapter 16.

Retained Deciduous Teeth

The time of shedding of deciduous teeth is quite variable. However, prolonged retention of a deciduous tooth may deflect the successor or prevent it from erupting. On the other hand, a deciduous tooth may be retained due to absence or misplacement of its successor.

Incisors

The roots of a deciduous incisor may fail to resorb if there is a periapical granuloma but sometimes the reasons are obscure. Usually the permanent incisor will be deflected lingually as it develops on the lingual aspect of the roots of the deciduous predecessor. Provided that the deciduous tooth is extracted before the permanent incisor reaches the occlusal level, spontaneous alignment can be expected. However, if an upper incisor (usually a central) is deflected so that it erupts into lingual occlusion with the lowers, appliance treatment to move it labially will be required (*see* Chapter 9 for appliance design).

Canines
These may be retained due to malposition of the successor. If the permanent canine cannot be removed into the line of the arch, it may be appropriate to retain the deciduous tooth. It will usually remain in place until the patient is over 30 years of age.

Molars
These teeth may be retained due to absence of their successors. However, retained roots can deflect the premolar. If a retained deciduous molar prevents the successor from erupting or deflects it, the deciduous molar should be extracted. Sometimes a retained deciduous molar will submerge.

Submerging Deciduous Molars (Fig. 10.7)
The lower second deciduous molars are most frequently involved and there may or may not be a successor. Submergence seems to be due to ankylosis of the roots with the alveolar bone. As the face grows, the adjacent teeth and alveolar bone continue to grow occlusally, leaving behind the ankylosed tooth which drops below the occlusal level and appears to become submerged. In the majority of cases, the ankylosis becomes resorbed before the submergence is marked and the tooth is shed normally. However, some teeth continue to submerge and become

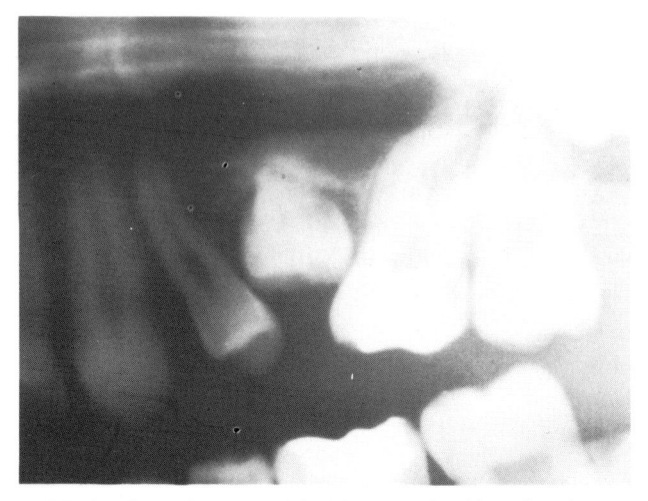

Fig. 10.7. A submerging second deciduous molar. Note that the second premolar is absent.

covered by alveolar mucosa. The adjacent teeth will tilt over the retained deciduous molar and quite a severe occlusal disharmony may result (*Fig.* 10.7). If a deciduous tooth is seen to be submerging, it is wise to keep it under observation to see whether it will become free and re-erupt to reach the occlusal level. If this does not happen and the submergence becomes more severe, the tooth should be carefully extracted. This may not be easy if the ankylosis is extensive. If there is no successor, appliance treatment to close the space may be neccessary (*see* p. 96).

Supernumerary teeth. Supernumerary teeth may be found in any region of the arch but they are particularly common adjacent to the upper midline (*Fig.* 10.8). Such a tooth, which is usually conical or tuberculate, is called a 'mesiodens'. Extra teeth may be found elsewhere in the mouth and may resemble teeth of the normal series. For example, extra teeth in the lateral incisor region may look like normal lateral incisors and occasionally an extra

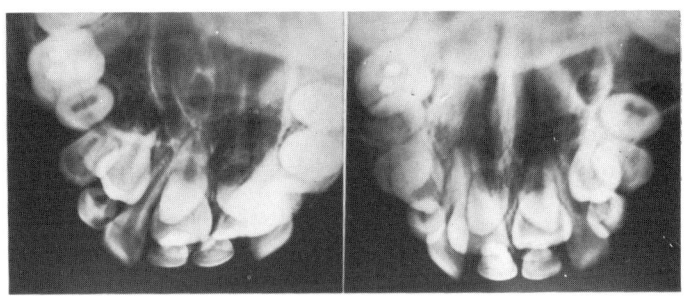

Fig. 10.8. Two radiographs showing the parallax method of determining the positions of two supernumerary teeth. The X-ray tube was moved a few inches between exposures. The supernumerary teeth appear to have moved in the same direction. This means that they are palatal to the roots of the central incisors.

premolar is found. Such teeth, resembling those of the normal series and developing where there has been an evolutionary reduction in the number of teeth (viz. the lateral incisor and premolar regions), are sometimes known as 'supplemental teeth'. In the molar region an extra peg-shaped tooth (sometimes known as a 'paramolar') may be found. It is usually buccal to a permanent molar and may be fused with it to give an extra buccal cusp. Occasionally a fourth molar may be present.

Patients with clefts of the lip and palate have a high prevalence of supernumerary teeth adjacent to the cleft (*see* Chapter 20).

Supernumerary teeth usually cause crowding and they should be extracted. Occasionally, where there is a supplemental lateral incisor, it is difficult to decide which is the tooth of the normal series and so the tooth in the less favourable position should be removed.

Mesiodens

These are quite commonly found (in about 1% of normal children). They may displace the permanent incisor, usually labially or distally, causing a median diastema; they may produce a rotation of the incisor; prevent eruption of the tooth; or they may have no clinical effect. A mesiodens may erupt and can be extracted simply, but many do not and it is necessary, before surgically removing them, to ascertain their relationship with the central incisors.

Investigation. Sometimes there are no clinical signs and the mesiodens is discovered on a routine radiograph. Where an upper central incisor is displaced, rotated or fails to erupt, an intra-oral film should always be taken to check whether one or more extra teeth are present. (A mesiodens is the commonest cause of failure of eruption of an upper central incisor.) Having confirmed the presence of a mesiodens, it is necessary to ascertain its relationship with the central incisor. Most of these teeth are palatal. Parallax views (*Fig.* 10.8) are the simplest method of locating the extra tooth. However, intra-oral views may give a misleading impression of the depth of the tooth and ideally a lateral skull film should be taken.

Treatment. Supernumerary teeth should be extracted. The only exception is the deeply buried mesiodens which is symptom-free and whose removal would endanger the vitality of the central incisors. If the permanent incisors have been displaced, their position may improve following the surgery but frequently appliances will be needed to align them.

Where the central incisor has been prevented from erupting, it is important that removal of the mesiodens is not delayed unduly, otherwise the adjacent permanent teeth may encroach upon the space. If this has happened, space must be regained first. Ideally, surgery should be undertaken shortly after the normal time of eruption of the permanent incisor (when about two-thirds of the root has formed). Details of surgery are discussed in Chapter 19. Following surgery and given adequate space, the central incisor may erupt normally. Should this not happen, perhaps because the incisor has become impacted against the root of the other central incisor, a bracket may be bonded to the tooth and very gentle traction applied to bring it into the line of the arch.

For convenience of reference, the causes of median diastema and of failure of eruption of a central incisor are listed below.

Median diastema

1. Physiological spacing (*see* p. 41).

2. Missing or peg-shaped lateral incisors (*see* p. 95).

3. Generalized spacing of the upper labial segment, possibly associated with proclination of the upper incisors.

4. A supernumerary tooth (*see* p. 111).

5. Abnormal labial fraenum (*see* p. 116).

6. Dilaceration of a central incisor (*see below*).

7. Rarely a median cyst.

Failure of eruption of a central incisor

1. A supernumerary tooth (*see* p. 111).

2. Dilaceration tooth (*see below*).

3. Scar tissue following surgical intervention (*see* p. 181).

4. Occasionally there may be no obvious cause and surgical exposure may be indicated.

ANOMALIES OF FORM AND POSITION

Anomalies of Form

Many anomalies of form are developmental: abnormally large teeth, peg-shaped teeth, geminations and *dens-in-dente* may all give rise to local malocclusions. Sometimes it is possible to adjust the form of the tooth (e.g. by crowning a peg lateral or removing an extra cusp, remembering that there may be an associated pulp horn) but often it will have to be extracted (e.g. a *dens-in-dente* in the upper lateral incisor region). In these cases, the treatment plan is designed either to close the space or to fill it with a prosthesis.

Dilaceration

This is the deformation of a tooth due to a disturbance during its normal formation as result of which the root is bent. It may occur in an impacted tooth where the root grows against and is deflected by a hard bony plate. For example, the roots of an impacted lower third molar may be deflected by the mandibular canal. Of greater orthodontic importance is the dilaceration of an upper incisor (usually the central) subsequent to the traumatic intrusion of a deciduous incisor most commonly in the 4–5 year old child. The already-formed portion of the tooth is displaced while the developing root continues to grow in the original direction. Where the dilaceration is only very slight, the tooth may erupt normally. It may be possible to align the crown by orthodontic appliances but the root position often precludes this; or it may be possible to crown the tooth. Where dilaceration is at all severe, the tooth will fail to erupt and in most cases will have to be extracted. A decision then has to be made whether to utilize the space or fit a prosthetic replacement (*see* p. 100).

Anomalies of Position

Many abnormal tooth positions reflect crowding. However, certain malpositions are developmental in origin: ectopic positions (often involving the upper permanent canine) and transpositions (usually involving either the upper canine and first premolar or lower canine and lateral incisor) must be attributed to abnormal developmental positions. Where the tooth is grossly misplaced, it will usually have to be extracted. Less severe malpositions frequently require fixed appliances to deal with them.

Upper permanent canines are among the most frequently malpositioned teeth. By the age of 8–10 years they should be palpable buccally. When this is not the case, their positions should be checked using parallax radiographs. If the permanent canine is palatally positioned, serious consideration should be given to extracting the no attempt should be made to control them at this stage. Should the habit persist into the period of the deciduous dentition, a malocclusion may result. This depends in part on the direction and duration of the forces applied by the thumb and in part on whether there are other factors which may contribute to the malocclusion (e.g. a Class II skeletal pattern and lack of lip seal). Typically there will be proclination of upper and retroclination of lower incisors giving an increase in overjet; depression of incisors to give an incomplete overbite or anterior open bite (often somewhat asymmetrical); and narrowing of the upper arch, due to contraction of the buccinator muscles, so that the arches are of equal width and there is lateral displacement of the mandible on closure (*see* p. 133).

If the habit is given up before the permanent incisors erupt, their positions will not be affected. However, a lateral displacement of the mandible may be perpetuated as the permanent teeth erupt and this must be treated.

The majority of children stop thumb sucking before 6 years of age. Some but not all the children in whom the habit persists will develop a malocclusion in the permanent dentition (*Fig.* 10.9). The factors determining whether a malocclusion will be produced are the same as those discussed above for the deciduous dentition, and the irregularity found is similar, viz. an increase in overjet, a reduction in overbite and possibly a narrowing of the upper arch so that there is a lateral displacement of the mandible and unilateral crossbite.

Where there is an incomplete overbite, the tongue will come forwards over the lower incisors during swallowing. This means that even if the habit is given up the malocclusion may not improve spontaneously.

If a child over 9 years of age persists in thumb sucking an attempt should be made to stop the habit. As a first step, encouragement should be tried and is often successful. Should this fail, and provided that the child is keen to stop, a simple removable appliance is often sufficient to break the habit. There must be no coercion but the

116   WALTHER'S ORTHODONTIC NOTES

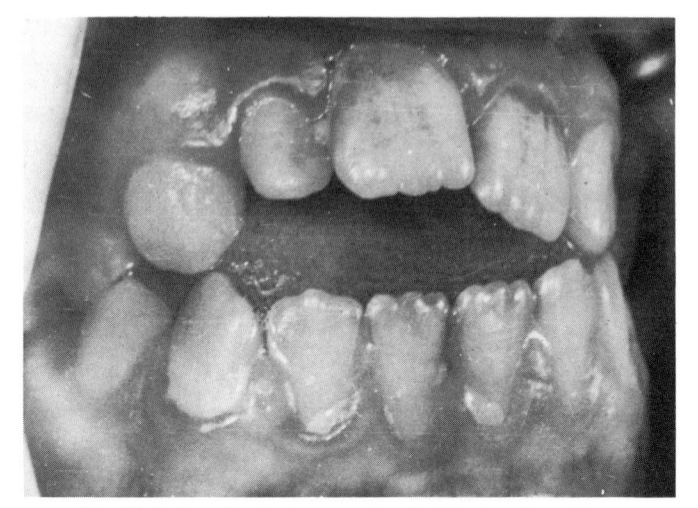

Fig. 10.9. A malocclusion associated with thumb sucking.

presence of the appliance makes the habit less satisfying. Children who fail to break the habit should be left until they are older and more mature. Nothing is to be gained by trying to force the issue.

Upper Labial Fraenum

In the infant the upper labial fraenum extends from the inner surface of lip, across the alveolar process to the palatine papilla. When the deciduous incisors erupt this continuity is normally lost and the fraenum becomes attached to the labial surface of the alveolar process. In a few children the fraenum will persist and this may be associated with a median diastema. Where there is a persistent fraenum, the palatine papilla will blanch if the lip is pulled forwards. It must be emphasized that although a persistent fraenum is often associated with a diastema, it is not a common cause and, in general, treatment should be withheld until the upper canines have erupted to see whether the space will close spontaneously. The causes of median diastema are listed on p. 113. Occasionally, if the fraenum is abnormally thick and fleshy, it will be a primary aetiological factor in producing a median diastema. In these cases a fraenectomy (Chapter 19) is indicated but if the diastema does not close spontaneously after surgery an appliance should be fitted.

Chapter 11

Tooth-Arch Disproportion

Disproportion between tooth size and arch size is common. It is usually manifest as crowding but occasionally there is generalized spacing. Tooth size is under direct genetic control while arch size depends on skeletal base size and on the soft tissue morphology and activity, both of which are under the influence of genetic factors.

SPACING

This is best accepted unless it gives an unsightly appearance in the upper labial segment. In this region, the spacing may be concentrated in the midline as a median diastema. It is sometimes possible to obtain an acceptable result by moving the upper central incisors together, distributing the space mesial and distal to the lateral incisors. A fraenectomy (Chapter 19) may then be performed and this will help to stabilize the result. If this is not done the diastema will frequently reopen. Sometimes, if the crowns of the lateral incisors are small, it is possible to build them up to mask the spaces.

Where spacing is more generalized and if treatment is indicated, appliances may be used to concentrate the spacing in the buccal segments, usually between the canine and first premolar. Some form of prosthesis (preferably a bridge) will then be required both for aesthetic reasons and to prevent relapse.

CROWDING

Crowding is common and any teeth may be involved: the incisors and canines if the arch is narrow or short; the

TOOTH-ARCH DISPROPORTION 119

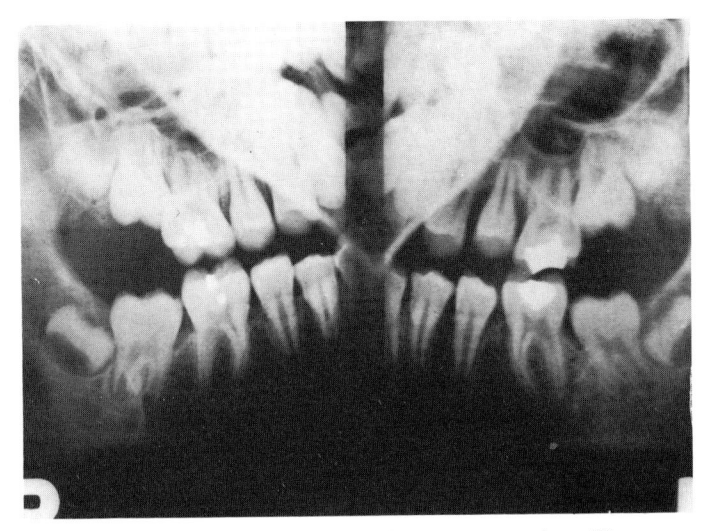

Fig. 11.1. Crowding in the upper and lower molar regions. The upper molars are 'stacked'. The lower third molars will be impacted.

molars where the arch is short (*see Fig.* 11.1); the premolars and canines if there had been drift of teeth following early loss of deciduous molars (*see Fig.* 10.1).

In general, it is not possible to produce a stable increase in arch size by labial movement of incisors or lateral expansion of buccal segments. Provided that the skeletal bases are long and the molars are not crowded, small amounts of space can sometimes be gained by distal movement of buccal segments using extra-oral traction (Chapter 9). However, if appreciable amounts of space are required to relieve crowding, extractions are required. Clearly the choice of extraction will be influenced by the poor conditon or abnormal form of any teeth. However, in the following discussion it will be assumed, unless explicitly stated otherwise, that all permanent teeth are present and sound.

Treatment of the upper and lower arches is discussed

separately. It is, of course, essential that treatment of the arches should be co-ordinated. This is discussed with the different classes of malocclusion (Chapters 13–16).

The Crowded Lower Arch

Crowded Incisors and Canines

Crowding is very common in this area and it tends to become worse with age, in part due to mesial drift of the buccal segments but more importantly due to the uprighting of the lower incisors which occurs during the later stages of facial growth. If the crowding is very mild and the lower arch is not crowded elsewhere, it may be best to accept the irregularity. However, if crowding is appreciable, extractions should be undertaken. Provided that the lower canines are mesially inclined, the extraction of lower first premolars will usually be followed by satisfactory spontaneous alignment of the labial segment. Any residual space will be taken up by forward drift of the buccal segments. Extractions are best undertaken after the lower canines have emerged through the alveolar mucosa but before they have reached the occlusal level. However, the lower canines commonly erupt before the first premolars and so this is not always possible. Should crowding be very severe so that most or all of the extraction space is required, a space maintainer should be fitted. Where the lower canines are distally inclined spontaneous resolution of lower incisor crowding will not follow the extraction of first premolars, and lower fixed appliance treatment to retract the canines is usually indicated. Where a lower canine is crowded it is sometimes tempting to extract this tooth. However, the approximal contact between a lower lateral incisor and first premolar is rarely satisfactory due to the shape of the teeth and so extraction of a lower canine should be avoided if possible.

Although it often seems to offer a simple solution to lower incisor crowding, normally the extraction of a lower incisor should be avoided for the following reasons:

1. Crowding frequently reappears among the remaining three incisors.

2. The lower intercanine width decreases and this may lead to a secondary reduction in upper intercanine width with crowding in the upper labial segment.

3. It is not possible to fit four upper incisors around three lower incisors: either an increase in overjet or upper incisor crowding may have to be accepted unless the upper canines can be retracted beyond their normal relationship with the lower canines.

However, in a few well-defined cases, listed below, the extraction of a lower incisor may be appropriate, although some of the problems mentioned above still apply:

1. Where one lower incisor is completely excluded from the arch and there are satisfactory approximal contacts between the other incisors.

2. Where one lower incisor is damaged (e.g. fractured) or where there is extensive periodontal recession so that its long term survival is in doubt. Fixed appliances are usually required to close the space.

3. Where one lower incisor is severely malpositioned so that appliance treatment would present problems. Fixed applicances are still usually necessary to achieve space closure and alignment of the other teeth.

4. Where the lower canines are severely distally inclined and the lower incisors are fanned there may be a case for extracting a lower incisor. However, alignment of the remaining incisors requires fixed appliance treatment and it is usually preferable in these cases to extract first premolars and use fixed appliances to retract and upright the canines.

Crowded Lower Premolars

Where there has been early loss of deciduous molars, space loss may follow so that the premolars are crowded. It will commonly be the second premolar which is short of space as it usually erupts later than the first. The second premolar may become impacted between the first premolar and first permanent molar or be deflected lingually. If space loss is slight and the second premolar erupts before the second permanent molar, it may force its way into the arch by driving the first molar distally or by forcing the anterior teeth mesially so that incisor crowding increases. Sometimes it is appropriate to fit a lower removable appliance to move the first molar distally (*see Fig.* 9.17). This may be undertaken more readily following extraction of the lower second permanent molar (*see below*).

In the majority of cases, space loss is moderate and there may also be crowding of the lower incisors. In these circumstances, extraction of the first premolar may be indicated. Extraction of the second premolar does not usually allow a satisfactory approximal contact between the first premolar and first permanent molar: the teeth tip towards one another and a stagnation area is created between them.

Where space loss has been severe so that there is already an approximal contact between the first premolar and first permanent molar, the extraction of the second premolar is advised. It should be remembered that the second premolar is slightly wider than the first and so extraction of the latter tooth will not give sufficient space. Severe space loss of the type mentioned above usually follows very early loss of the second deciduous molar, allowing the first permanent molar to erupt too far forward. In these circumstances, the first permanent molar is reasonably upright and an acceptable approximal contact with the first premolar is present.

Crowded Lower Molars

Impaction of lower first or second permanent molars is rare and probably reflects an abnormal developmental position of the tooth rather than crowding. However, crowding of third molars is very common and, unless other permanent teeth are missing or have been extracted, there is rarely room to accommodate them in the arch. If the lower arch is otherwise regular, the extraction of the crowded third molar itself is the most suitable treatment. This should be undertaken either by a lateral approach at the time of crown completion (*see* Chapter 19) or by conventional surgical techniques when about two-thirds of the roots have formed. It is not wise to ignore crowded third molars until they give trouble because—

1. They are more difficult to remove when the roots are completed.

2. If pericoronitis develops, a periodontal pocket may be produced on the distal aspect of the lower second permanent molar.

3. In a few cases, their eruptive force may contribute to mesial drift of the buccal segments, producing crowding elsewhere.

Extraction of lower second permanent molars to provide space for crowded third molars is not usually indicated because the position of eruption of the third molar is variable and it will rarely come into as good a position as the second molar originally occupied. However, where a small amount of space is also required in the second premolar region or where the second permanent molar is extensively carious, its removal may be indicated. Timing is important. For the best results (*Fig.* 11.2), the second molar should be removed just after root formation of the third molar has started, usually between 12 and 14 years of age. It is important that the third molar is in a favourable position: it should be slightly mesially inclined, its long axis forming an angle of less than $30°$ to the long axis of the second molar. However, as mentioned above, although the timing of extraction of the second molar is correct and the position of the third molar is favourable, it is not possible to guarantee a good result.

First permanent molars are never the teeth of choice for orthodontic extraction. However, where one or more of

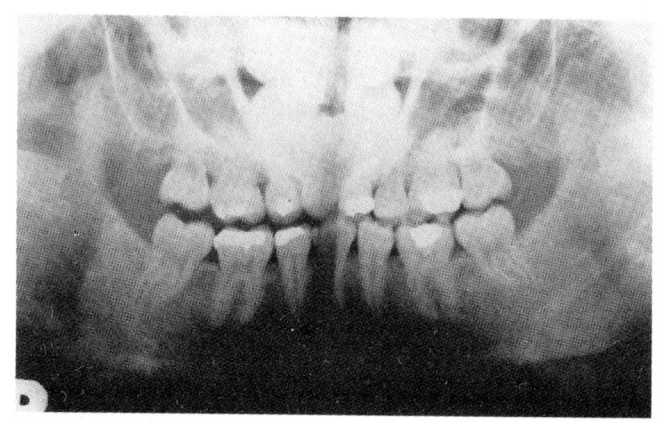

Fig. 11.2. In this case, the extraction of second molars has allowed the third molars to erupt into a good position.

these teeth are extensively carious their removal must be considered. This has been discussed on pp. 106–108.

The Crowded Upper Arch

Crowded Incisors and Canines

As in the case of the lower arch and provided that the canines are mesially inclined, extraction of first premolars usually gives the most satisfactory result. For maximal spontaneous improvement of crowding, the first premolars should be extracted after the canines have emerged into the mouth but before they have reached the occlusal level. They should not be retracted with an appliance until they have reached the occlusal level. Care should be taken to ensure that forward drift of the buccal segments does not encroach on the space required for the canines. If space is short a space maintainer should be fitted.

Sometimes in crowded cases, there is a good approximal contact between the permanent upper lateral incisor and first premolar with the canine completely excluded from the arch. In these cases, extraction of the canine should be considered. The upper canine is slightly wider than the first premolar and extraction of the premolar will not provide sufficient space to accommodate the canine. If the canine is distally inclined or palatally placed and it is possible to obtain a satisfactory contact between the lateral incisor and first premolar by simple orthodontic treatment, extraction of the canine should again be considered. To improve the appearance it may be necessary to grind down the palatal cusp of the first premolar. A problem arises if the first premolar is mesiobuccally rotated because the appearance is then rather poor. In these circumstances fixed appliance treatment may be required, either to align the premolar after extraction of the canine or to align the canine following extraction of the premolar. The treatment of choice depends on the features of the individual case.

If a lateral incisor is crowded into lingual occlusion with the apex palatally displaced and if the canine is erupting in a forward position and is upright or distally inclined, consideration may be given to extraction of the lateral incisor itself. The presence of a canine adjacent to a central incisor does not usually give an ideal appearance and, where possible, it is preferable to extract the first premolar or the canine to provide space for the lateral incisor. However, fixed appliance treatment would be required to move the lateral incisor apex forward. If the patient is unsuitable for or is unwilling to wear fixed appliances, the simple expedient of extracting the lateral incisor may be justified.

Crowded Upper Premolars

As in the case of the lower arch, it is usually the second premolar which is crowded. If there is a good approximal contact between the first premolar and first permanent molar, the second premolar should be extracted. However, where the first premolar and first permanent molar are not in contact and particularly if there is also incisor or canine crowding, the first premolar should be removed to make space for the alignment of the second premolar. Where crowding is very mild, it may be possible to make space for the crowded second premolar by moving back the first permanent molar with an appliance possibly following extraction of the second permanent molar (*see below*).

Crowded Upper Permanent Molars

In the developing dentition, crowding of the upper molars will be manifest as 'stacking' (*see Fig.* 11.1). When they erupt crowded molars are usually distally and buccally inclined.

Impaction of upper first permanent molars against the second deciduous molars is a result of their abnormal developmental position rather than crowding. First permanent molars are not the teeth of choice for orthodontic extraction. Treatment planning, where the extraction of these teeth is necessitated because of their poor life expectancy, is discussed on pp. 106–108.

It is usually the third permanent molars which are crowded and if the arch is otherwise well aligned these teeth should be extracted on eruption. If more space is required to allow retraction of the upper buccal segments and provided that third molars are present, of normal size and in favourable positions, upper second molars may be extracted. In contrast with the lower arch, the third molar will usually erupt to obtain a satisfactory contact relationship with the first permanent molar.

Serial Extractions

This is a procedure where, in order to encourage the spontaneous alignment of crowded incisors, the timely removal of certain deciduous and permanent teeth is undertaken.

1. The four deciduous canines are removed as the upper permanent lateral incisors are erupting (at about $8\frac{1}{2}$ years of age); the alignment of the incisors should improve at the expense of space for the permanent canines.

2. The first deciduous molars are removed in order to encourage the early eruption of the first premolars. This will be most successful if the premolar roots have half formed (at about $9\frac{1}{2}$ years of age). It is desirable that the first premolars should erupt in advance of the canines although this is often not the case in the lower arch.

3. When the upper permanent canines have just emerged through the oral mucosa, the first premolars should be extracted. This is the most important stage of serial extraction procedure and it is essential to recheck that the case is suitable for treatment by extraction of first premolars: all teeth must be present and sound; the permanent canines must be mesially inclined; and there must be crowding sufficient to justify the extraction of first premolars. If these conditions do not apply the case must be treated on its merits: the fact that serial extractions have been started by removal of deciduous canines does not commit one to going through with this line of treatment.

The full serial extraction procedure has several disadvantages: the child is subjected to extractions on a number of occasions; the lower permanent canine may erupt ahead of the first premolar into the extraction space of the first deciduous molar, impacting the premolar and making its removal difficult; and, quite frequently, the patient requires appliance treatment anyway.

In spite of the disadvantages and limitations of serial extractions as a technique, the principle of timing extractions to take advantage of spontaneous tooth movements is still valid: the removal of deciduous canines to allow spontaneous alignment of crowded incisors may simplify later appliance treatment; and the extraction of a first premolar before a crowded, mesially inclined canine has fully erupted allows it to drift into the line of the arch without appliance treatment. However, there is seldom any advantage to be gained from the extraction of first deciduous molars in order to encourage the eruption of the first premolars.

Chapter 12

Arch Malrelationships

Arch malrelationships may occur in any plane. Antero-posterior arch malrelationships are the basis of Angles classification as described in Chapter 6.

ANTERO-POSTERIOR MALRELATIONSHIPS
Buccal Segments

Antero-posterior malrelationships of the buccal segments often reflect antero-posterior jaw malrelationships but, because the position of the teeth in relation to the skeletal base can vary, it is possible to find cases with normal skeletal relationships and arch malrelationships, and vice versa. When the lower buccal segment is posteriorly positioned relative to the upper, this may be referred to as a Class II buccal segment relationship or as a disto-occlusion; and where the lower buccal segment is forward in relation to the upper, this is a Class III buccal segment relationship or mesio-occlusion.

Labial Segments

The labial segment relationship often but not always follows the buccal segment relationship. For example it is possible to find a case with a Class II incisor relationship but a Class I or even Class III buccal segment relationship.

The aetiology and treatment of the different antero-posterior arch malrelationships are discussed in Chapters 13–16.

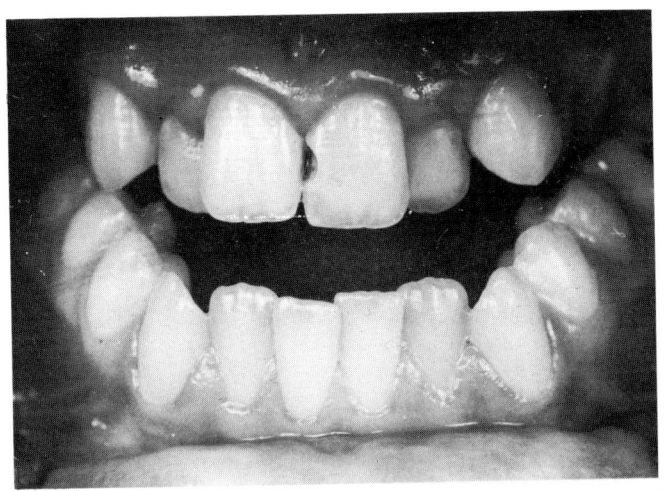

Fig. 12.1. This patient has a Class III malocclusion with a skeletal anterior open bite and a bilateral crossbite. These occlusal malrelationships reflect skeletal malrelationships: there is a Class III skeletal pattern; the lower facial third is increased in height; and the maxilla is narrow relative to the mandible.

VERTICAL MALRELATIONSHIPS

Buccal Segments

Vertical malrelationships are not common in the buccal segments.

Where the intermaxillary height is increased and there is a skeletal anterior open bite (*Fig.* 12.1) this may extend into the buccal segments so that perhaps only the most posterior molar teeth are in occlusion. In these cases there is a lateral open bite as well as an anterior open bite. Occasionally a lateral open bite is found in isolation from any other occlusal anomaly. The reasons for this are usually obscure but there may be a localized failure of alveolar development.

Over-eruption of buccal teeth which are unopposed is of course seen quite commonly.

Labial Segments

In normal occlusion the lower incisors occlude with the cingulum plateau of the upper incisors and the overbite is one-third to one-half of the height of the lower incisor crowns.

Increase in Overbite

Skeletal factors. It is often stated that a small lower facial height is associated with a deep overbite. However, this is not a constant relationship and occlusal factors (*see below*) must also play a part.

Occlusal factors. Where there is no incisor contact due to a large overjet (Class II division 1), the lower incisors will often erupt until they contact the palatal mucosa and the overbite will be deep. Where there is an adaptive anterior oral seal between tongue and lower lip, the overbite is incomplete but is still deep in most cases (Chapter 3).

Where the overjet is normal and the upper incisors are retroclined (Class II division 2), so that the inter-incisor angle is increased, the overbite will also be increased. This may happen developmentally or as a result of treatment of a severe Class II division 1 incisor relationship with removable appliances so that the upper incisors are over-retroclined (*see Fig.* 14.3). Even if the overbite has been reduced during treatment, it will increase again when appliances are discarded.

The reduction of a deep overbite will be stable only if at the end of treatment the lower incisors occlude with the palatal surfaces of the upper incisors; the inter-incisor angle is within normal range; and the teeth are in a position of labiolingual balance.

Reduction in Overbite

If there is a mild Class III incisor relationship with occlusion between the upper and lower incisors, the overbite will be reduced.

An overbite may be reduced and incomplete for a

variety of reasons which are dealt with below under 'Anterior Open Bite'.

Anterior Open Bite

Here there is no occlusal contact between the incisors, and the upper incisors do not overlap the lowers in the vertical plane. Anterior open bite is discussed below according to its aetiology: skeletal, soft tissue, habit and miscellaneous.

Skeletal factors. Where the anterior intermaxillary space is increased, the vertical growth of the labial segments may be insufficient to achieve tooth contact when the posterior teeth are brought into occlusion (*Fig.* 12.1). In the most severe cases only the last standing teeth will meet in occlusion. Generally, the Frankfort mandibular planes angle is increased and frequently, but not always, there is a Class III skeletal pattern.

It is interesting that except in the most severe cases, the open bite is seldom of concern to the patient either aesthetically or functionally. Frequently, of course, coexisting features such as mandibular protrusion do worry the patient. Correction of the anterior open bite is rarely indicated: orthodontic treatment to elongate the incisors will rarely be successful; extraction or grinding of posterior teeth is definitely contraindicated because the patient will then be forced to overclose into occlusion, exaggerating any prominence of the mandible and possibly giving rise to muscle pain at a later date; overlay dentures are contraindicated because of the problems of food stagnation and because they rarely improve the appearance of this type of patient. The only successful treatment is surgery (*see* Chapter 19) but this should not be done unless the patient is particularly concerned. Of course, if surgery to correct a Class III skeletal pattern is to be undertaken it should be planned to deal with the open bite at the same time.

Soft tissue factors. Where there is an anterior open bite due to other aetiological factors (e.g. a habit) the tongue will frequently come forwards to fill the gap. This is a purely adaptive behaviour. A tongue-to-lip anterior oral seal (*see* Chapter 3) is usually associated with an incomplete overbite. The tongue behaviour will readapt on correction of the overbite. In the rare cases of primary atypical tongue thrust, the soft tissue activity is responsible for an incomplete overbite or even an anterior open bite. As discussed in Chapter 3, these cases are not suitable for orthodontic treatment.

Habits. Thumb or finger sucking may produce an anterior open bite (*see Fig.* 10.9) which will often improve on cessation of the habit.

Miscellaneous. The various developmental (e.g. cleft palate), pathological (e.g. bony dysplasia) and traumatic (e.g. bilateral condylar fracture) causes of anterior open bite will not be discussed here. Generally the open bite is only a minor feature of the condition and is not the primary cause of concern.

TRANSVERSE MALRELATIONSHIPS

Buccal Segments

A transverse malrelationship of the buccal segments is termed a 'crossbite' and this may be bilateral (*Fig.* 12.1) or unilateral (*Fig.* 12.2). In most cases of crossbite the upper arch is narrow relative to the lower so that the buccal cusps of the lower teeth overlap the buccal cusps of the uppers. Occasionally, a lingual crossbite or scissors bite is found in which the upper teeth completely overlap the lowers buccally.

Bilateral Crossbite

This is a symmetrical transverse arch malrelationship and is usually skeletal in origin. The maxilla is narrow in relation to the mandible and this is reflected in the arch widths. Bilateral crossbites are frequently found in association with severe Class III malocclusions (*see Fig.*

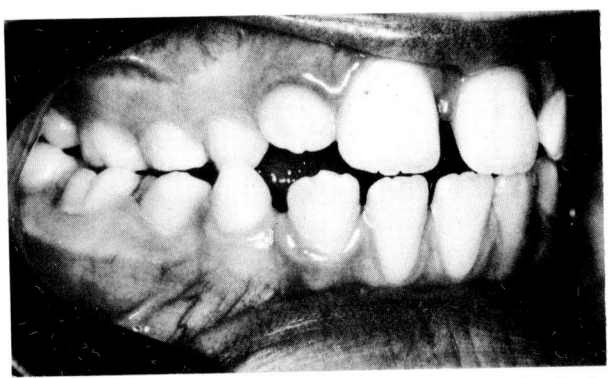

Fig. 12.2. A unilateral crossbite. Note that the lower centre line is also off to the right. In centric relation this patient's buccal teeth would meet cusp to cusp, and so there is a lateral displacement to the right in order to obtain maximal occlusion.

12.1), in part because the maxilla is often narrow relative to the mandible and in part because a broader part of the lower arch opposes a narrower part of the upper arch.

Although from a theoretical viewpoint masticatory efficiency is reduced, in practice a bilateral crossbite is seldom of functional significance. Additionally, expansion of the upper arch to correct the crossbite is rarely stable. Thus these malocclusions are usually best left untreated. Occasionally rapid expansion of the mid-palatal suture may be attempted using a fixed appliance. This should be undertaken only as part of a more general treatment plan and, although expansion of the suture may be stable, occlusal relapse may still follow.

Unilateral Crossbite

It is important to distinguish between unilateral crossbites with lateral displacement and those without.

With displacement (*Fig.* 12.2). In most non-pathological cases of unilateral crossbite, when the mandible is at rest, the arches are symmetrical. However, both arches have the same relative width and with normal hinge closure the cheek teeth would meet cusp to cusp. In order to achieve maximal intercuspation, the mandible is displaced to one side so that there is an apparently asymmetrical malocclusion. Generally, the midlines of the arches will be coincident at rest, but in occlusion the lower midline will be displaced to the side of the crossbite.

The aetiology of this type of occlusion may be a transverse skeletal discrepancy similar to but less severe than the type causing a bilateral crossbite (i.e. the maxilla may be narrow relative to the mandible and there may be a mild Class III skeletal pattern). However, a unilateral crossbite of this type may be caused by soft tissue factors. For example, if swallowing habitually takes place without occlusion of the teeth, pressure from the cheeks may equalize the widths of the arches. Similarly with habits such as persistent thumb sucking, forces from the cheeks while the teeth are not in occlusion may narrow the maxillary arch so that a unilateral crossbite with mandibular displacement occurs.

The amount of expansion of the upper arch necessary to correct the crossbite is small and, unlike a bilateral crossbite, the occlusion of the teeth will normally prevent relapse. As the maxillary arch is basically symmetrical the expansion should be bilateral.

Without displacement. Here there is a true asymmetry of one arch which will often reflect an underlying skeletal asymmetry. This may be within normal limits but occasionally it is produced by some pathological factor (e.g. unilateral cleft palate produces a maxillary asymmetry, while unilateral condylar hyperplasia may produce a mandibular asymmetry with secondary occlusal effects).

Clearly, where the crossbite is produced by some pathological factor, treatment considerations will primarily be directed towards the basic anomaly although occlusal factors are also important. (Cleft palate is discussed in Chapter 20.) A unilateral crossbite without displacement in a normal individual does not usually require treatment but, if treatment is undertaken, it may be unstable.

Chapter 13

Class I Malocclusions

OCCLUSAL FEATURES

Class I includes those malocclusions where there is a normal sagittal arch relationship (*see Fig.* 6.1, p. 48). There may be local malocclusions such as those produced by dental anomalies; crowding or spacing; or lateral or vertical malrelationships between the arches. These have already been discussed in Chapters 10–12.

LABIAL SEGMENTS

In a Class I incisor relationship, the lower incisor edges should occlude with or lie directly below the cingulum plateau of the upper incisors (*Fig.* 13.1). This relationship need not apply to all the incisors: for example, there may be local irregularities such as rotations or there may be one or two instanding upper incisors. However, taking the labial segments, as a whole, there should be a normal antero-posterior relationship between them.

SKELETAL RELATIONSHIPS

Antero-posterior

The skeletal pattern is usually Class I (*Fig.* 13.1) but it is possible to find a Class I malocclusion in association with a Class II or Class III skeletal pattern providing that the inclinations of the teeth, and their positions on the skeletal bases, compensate for the skeletal malrelationship.

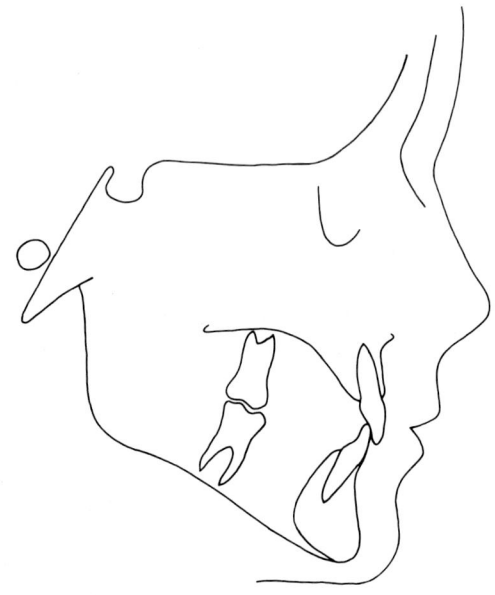

Fig. 13.1. A Class I malocclusion associated with a Class I skeletal pattern.

Vertical and Transverse

The jaw relationships in the vertical and transverse planes are usually within the normal range but there may be malrelationships in these planes and associated occlusal anomalies.

SOFT TISSUES

As in the case of the skeletal relationships, the soft tissue form and activity are usually within the normal range.

TREATMENT

The various local anomalies which may be present in Class I malocclusions have already been discussed under relevant headings in Chapter 10 and the appliances used have been described in Chapter 9.

Treatment Planning

Treatment of the upper and lower arches must be co-ordinated. As a rule, it is simplest to plan treatment of the lower arch first, then to build the upper arch around the lower.

The Lower Arch

The size and form of the lower arch must be accepted if the result is to be stable. Thus treatment to relieve crowding involves the extraction of teeth. If the crowding is moderate to severe and given that all teeth (apart from third molars) are present, sound and in favourable positions, the extraction of first premolars is usually indicated. This has been discussed at greater length in Chapter 11. Usually spontaneous alignment of the teeth will follow the extractions provided that these are undertaken while the occlusion is developing and the canines are mesially inclined.

The Upper Arch

As a general rule in Class I cases, if extractions are necessary in the lower arch, teeth (usually first premolars) should be removed from the upper arch. This will then provide adequate space to align the upper arch and achieve correct occlusal relationships with the lower arch. Details of treatment planning are discussed in Chapter 11 and appliances in Chapter 9.

Chapter 14

Class II Division 1 Malocclusions

OCCLUSAL FEATURES

According to Angle's classification, the lower arch should be at least one-half cusp width postnormal to the upper, and there is an increase in overjet (*see Fig.* 6.2). It should be remembered that it is only the relationship between the dental arches that is taken into account in classification and it is not necessarily the lower arch which is at fault in Class II cases: the upper arch may be too far forward in the facial complex.

LABIAL SEGMENTS

The upper incisors are usually proclined but may be of average inclination. The lower labial segment shows no characteristic features: it is often crowded but may be spaced; the lower incisors may be proclined or retroclined, depending on the soft tissue pattern.

The incisor relationship is Class II division 1: the lower incisor edges lie posterior to the cingulum plateau of the upper incisors and there is an increase in overjet (*Fig.* 14.1).

The overbite is usually deep. It may be complete but is often slightly incomplete if there is a tongue-to-lower-lip anterior oral seal (*Fig.* 14.2). Sometimes the overbite is quite markedly incomplete, perhaps due to a thumb-sucking habit or occasionally as a result of a primary atypical swallowing pattern.

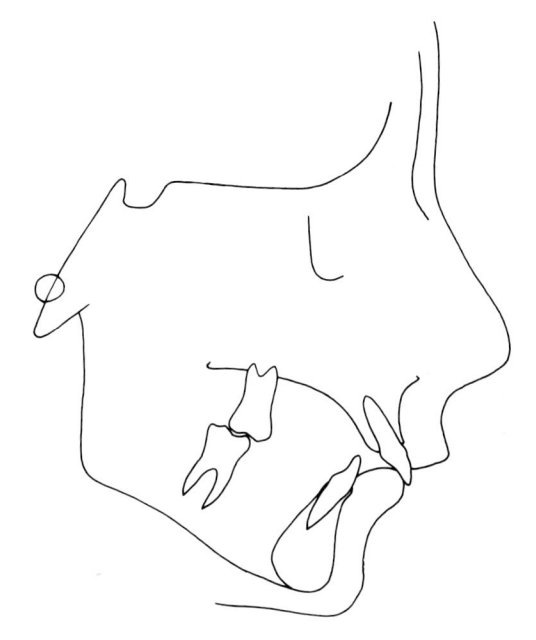

Fig. 14.1. A Class II division 1 malocclusion associated with a Class II skeletal pattern.

SKELETAL RELATIONSHIPS
Antero-posterior

There is usually a Class II skeletal pattern (*Fig.* 14.1). In many cases this is the primary aetiological factor responsible for the Class II arch relationship. The more severe the skeletal malrelationship, the more severe the malocclusion is likely to be and the poorer the prognosis for treatment. Sometimes, due to the soft tissue pattern, the inclination of the lower teeth will to some extent compensate for the skeletal pattern: the lower incisors may be proclined and thus the overjet will be less than might have been expected.

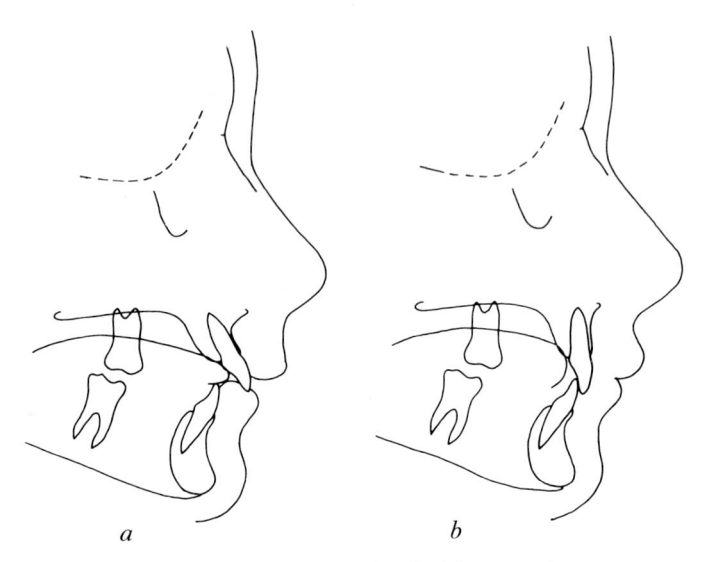

Fig. 14.2. *a*, An adaptive anterior oral seal with contact between tongue and lower lip. *b*, Following retraction of the upper incisors, an anterior seal will be obtained by lip contact. The lower lip covers the incisal third of the upper incisors and this will ensure stability of the overjet reduction.

In a number of cases the skeletal pattern is Class I (or rarely mild Class III). In these cases, it is the position of the teeth on the skeletal bases that is at fault, due either to their developmental positions or to their inclination under the influence of the soft tissues.

Vertical

The Frankfort mandibular plane angle is usually average or high. A high angle is regarded as an unfavourable feature, partly because the lips are more likely to be incompetent and partly because the lower incisors may be retroclined, exaggerating the overjet.

Transverse

There are no characteristic transverse malrelationships.

MANDIBULAR POSITIONS AND PATHS OF CLOSURE

In many cases the mandible is habitually in the rest position and there is a centric path of closure. In a few cases the mandible is habitually postured forwards to facilitate the production of a lip seal. In these cases an upwards and backwards deviation of the mandible on closure will be observed. True distal displacements are rare.

SOFT TISSUES

The lips are frequently incompetent. This often contributes to the lack of control and consequent proclination of the upper incisors. In some cases, a lip seal will be maintained but frequently, there is a tongue-to-lower-lip seal with the lower lip lying behind the upper incisors (*Fig.* 14.2). If, after retraction of the upper incisors, a lip seal will be obtained with the lower lip covering the incisal third of the upper incisor (*Fig.* 14.2), the outlook for stability is good. If, however, the lower lip does not control the corrected upper incisor position but a tongue-to-lower-lip anterior oral seal continues, the prognosis for treatment stability is poor.

In mild cases where a lip seal is obtained, the swallowing pattern will be normal. In more severe cases where there is a tongue-to-lower-lip seal, there will be an adaptive type of swallowing behaviour.

In a very few patients, there is a primary atypical swallowing behaviour (Chapter 3). This will be an aetiological factor in producing the incisor malrelationship and will preclude a stable reduction of the overjet. In these cases the overjet should be accepted.

HABITS

There is often a history of thumb sucking. In some cases, this may have contributed to the incisor malrelationship.

ORAL HEALTH

The incidence of fracture of upper incisors is higher in Class II division 1 cases. A hyperplastic gingivitis around the upper incisors is also common in Class II division 1 cases with habitually parted lips, due to drying of the exposed gingivae. This is sometimes incorrectly called a 'mouth-breathing gingivitis' although in fact these patients are not usually mouth breathers (there is often an anterior oral seal between tongue and lower lip and a posterior seal between the soft palate and dorsum of the tongue).

Even although in some cases with a deep, complete overbite the lower incisors occlude directly with the palatal mucosa, trauma is surprisingly rare.

TREATMENT

The primary objectives of treatment are to relieve crowding and to correct the incisor relationship. Attention should also be paid to the buccal segment relationship. In the interests of stability and occlusal function there should be a good intercuspation between the upper and lower teeth. A Class II buccal segment relationship (which may result if premolar extractions are undertaken only in the upper arch) is perfectly acceptable provided that the intercuspation is good.

Treatment Planning

The following discussion is based on the assumption that all teeth (except for third molars) are present, sound and in favourable positions.

The Lower Arch

The lower arch should be planned first. The form and size of the lower arch should be accepted and treatment confined to relief of crowding and alignment of teeth.

Where the lower arch is regular, no treatment is indicated. If there is crowding of a degree which warrants treatment extractions must be undertaken. The treatment of crowding has been discussed in detail in Chapter 11. The teeth most frequently selected for extraction are the lower first premolars. Provided that canines are mesially inclined and the extractions are undertaken while the occlusion is developing, satisfactory spontaneous alignment in the lower arch is to be expected.

The Upper Arch

Distal movement of buccal segments. Where the space requirements in the upper arch are mild (no more than 3 mm, i.e. less than one-half cusp width) and where the lower arch is well aligned (and no extractions are indicated except perhaps for lower second or third molars), distal movement of the upper buccal segments may be the best approach to treatment. The upper buccal segments must be well aligned. It is important that the first permanent molars are not already distally inclined. If there is 'stacking' of second and third molars (*see Fig.* 11.1), the extraction of the second permanent molars will provide space for and facilitate the retraction of the buccal segments. It is obviously essential that upper third molars are present and of normal size.

The buccal segments should be retracted until they are in a normal relationship with the lower arch. This should allow a correct intercuspation of the upper canines and so provide space for retraction of the upper labial segment. Following distal movement of the upper buccal segments, retraction of the canines may be required if they have not spontaneously followed the other buccal teeth. Retraction of the upper incisors will then be necessary. It is important that the anchorage for these tooth movements should be reinforced by extra-oral anchorage because the recently retracted buccal segments do not have a high anchorage value.

Retraction of canines. Space for retraction of the canines may have been provided by distal movement of the buccal segments as described above. Where an appreciable amount of space (more than 3 mm on each side) is required in the upper arch or where premolars have been extracted in the lower arch, removal of the upper first premolars is usually indicated (provided that the canines are mesially inclined). If this provides more space than is required, the buccal segments will normally drift forwards to close the gap after appliances have been discontinued. In severe cases where the extraction of upper first premolars provides only just sufficient space for full retraction of the upper canines into the correct relationship with the lower arch, extra-oral anchorage must be used to reinforce the intra-oral anchorage, particularly during the retraction of the canines. The upper canines should be retracted until they are in a correct relationship with the lower canines. If lower premolars are to be extracted, the upper canines should be retracted far enough to allow for any distal drift of the lower canines so that the upper incisors may be fully retracted.

Overbite reduction. If the overbite is deep it will have to be reduced prior to correction of the overjet and a flat anterior bite plane should be incorporated in the appliance at the canine retraction stage. This also has the advantage that it prevents occlusal interference with the canine retraction.

Retraction of the incisors. Provided that the lower arch is not crowded and the upper canines occlude in the embrasure distal to the lowers, there should be sufficient space to align the upper incisors around the lowers with a normal overbite and overjet. If the lower incisors are crowded, or if the upper canines have not been retracted far enough, it will be necessary to accept either upper incisor crowding or an increase in overjet.

CLASS II DIVISION 1 MALOCCLUSIONS 145

In planning treatment it is important to recognize that the upper incisors will be tipped about a point close to the middle of the root. If the incisors are already proclined and the overjet is not too large, it will be possible to reduce the overjet without the incisors becoming retroclined. If, however, the overjet is large or the upper incisors are not proclined, they will become unduly retroclined following retraction with a removable appliance. This conversion of a Class II division 1 into a Class II division 2 incisor relationship (*Fig.* 14.3) is undesirable both from an aesthetic point of view and because, if the inter-incisor angle is too large, the overbite will deepen following treatment. These cases should not be treated with removable appliances but, where possible, should be referred for treatment with fixed appliances which can bodily retract the upper incisors.

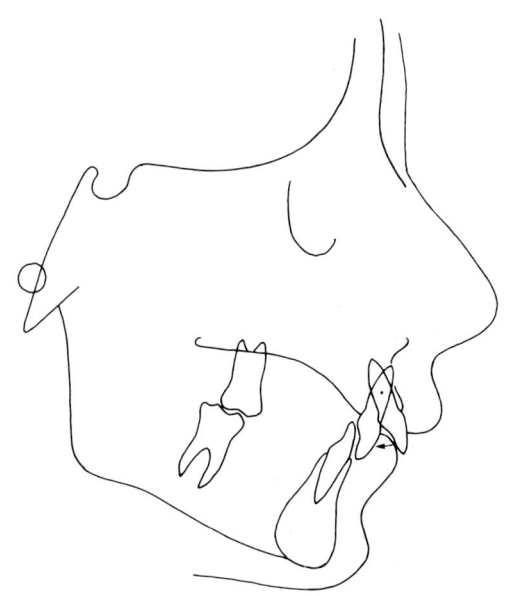

Fig. 14.3. When the overjet is large and if the upper incisors are not sufficiently proclined, retraction with a removable appliance will produce a Class II division 2 incisor relationship.

Stability

Following retraction, the upper incisors should be retained by an appliance for about 6 months to allow the supporting tissues to become fully readjusted to the new tooth positions.

Stability of overjet reduction depends on control of the upper incisors by the lower lip. If the lips are habitually held apart even after reduction of the overjet the case may relapse. Equally, in rare cases of primary tongue thrust, relapse will follow overjet reduction. These cases should, of course, be recognized at diagnosis, and treatment to reduce the overjet should not be undertaken.

As mentioned above, overbite stability depends on establishing a correct occlusal relationship between upper and lower incisors: if the overjet does relapse, the overbite will also increase; if the inter-incisor angle is too wide (greater than 145°) the overbite will deepen even though the overjet does not materially increase.

Chapter 15

Class II Division 2 Malocclusions

OCCLUSAL FEATURES
According to Angle's classification, the lower arch should be at least one-half cusp width postnormal to the upper, and the upper central incisors are retroclined (*see Fig.* 6.3).

Labial Segments

The amount of retroclination of the upper central incisors is closely related to the degree of postnormality of the lower arch which is, in turn, related to the severity of the skeletal malrelationship. The upper lateral incisors are often proclined, mesially inclined and mesiolabially rotated (*see Fig.* 6.3). Sometimes they are retroclined in line with the central incisors. The lower labial segment is often slightly crowded and the lower incisors may be retroclined, a feature which increases the inter-incisor angle and so has an adverse effect on the depth of overbite.

The overjet is usually only slightly increased, the distal position of the lower arch being compensated for by the retroclination of the upper central incisors. In severe cases where there is a marked Class II skeletal pattern, the overjet may be increased. The overbite is deep and complete, the depth of overbite depending on the severity of the skeletal malrelationship and on the size of the inter-incisor angle. The overbite may be only slightly increased but it is occasionally very deep with the lower incisors occluding on the palatal mucosa and the upper incisors on the gingivae labial to the lower incisors. Fortunately, for they are very difficult to treat, these severe cases are quite rare. The majority of Class II division 2 cases are mild with a deep but not excessive overbite.

Buccal Segments

These may be crowded if there has been early loss of deciduous molar teeth with forward drift of the first permanent molars.

SKELETAL RELATIONSHIPS

Antero-posterior

The skeletal pattern is usually Class I or mild Class II (*Fig.* 15.1). The profile is frequently well balanced, with the chin in a good relationship with the rest of the face.

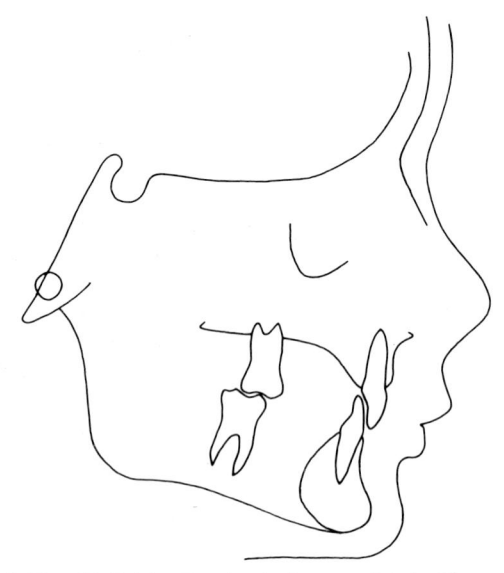

Fig. 15.1. A Class II division 2 malocclusion associated with a mild Class II skeletal pattern.

The receding chin so often seen in Class II division 1 cases is not common in Class II division 2. These malocclusions are not usually associated with severe Class II skeletal patterns unless the malocclusion is a result of treatment when the upper incisors in a severe Class II division 1 case have been tipped back to reduce the overjet (*see Fig.* 14.3).

Vertical

The lower facial height is reduced or average. The Frankfort mandibular planes angle is often low. The low anterior facial height may contribute to the depth of overbite.

Transverse

There are no characteristic malrelationships.

MANDIBULAR POSITIONS AND PATHS OF CLOSURE

In many cases, the habitual position of the mandible is the rest position and the path of closure into occlusion is a simple hinge movement. In some of the more severe cases, however, the mandible is habitually postured downwards and forwards. The reasons for this are obscure but it is important to recognize that the upwards and backwards path of closure in these cases is a deviation into a position of centric occlusion and is not a distal displacement. True posterior displacements are sometimes found in Class II division 2 cases, particularly where there has been loss of posterior teeth. These patients will often present with pain in early adult life. Attrition facets will be observed on certain teeth. Careful occlusal analysis and equilibration are necessary.

SOFT TISSUES

The lips are held together, usually with minimal circumoral contraction. The lip line is often high, the lower lip covering more than the occlusal half of the upper incisors. Variations in swallowing behaviour are not important in the aetiology or treatment of this malocclusion.

ORAL HEALTH

Oral health is usually good, given good oral hygiene and dental care. In cases with excessive overbite, where the lower incisors occlude with the palatal mucosa and the upper incisors with the gingivae labial to the lower incisors, direct trauma to the gingivae may develop. This often does not arise until the patient reaches adult life and is much more common where there has been loss of posterior teeth. An excessive overbite is a potentially traumatic relationship; it should where possible be corrected in the early permanent dentition. This is not easy and requires complex fixed appliance treatment.

TREATMENT

The objectives of treatment are as follows.
1. To relieve crowding and align the teeth.
2. If the overbite is excessive, to reduce it. Where the overbite is not excessively deep and there is tooth-to-tooth contact, it may be best to accept the position of the upper central incisors and to concentrate on aligning the other teeth. If the overbite has to be reduced, the inter-incisor angle must also be reduced by torquing back the upper incisor apices with fixed appliances.

Treatment Planning

It is of course essential to check that all teeth are present,

CLASS II DIVISION 2 MALOCCLUSIONS 151

Treatment Planning

It is of course essential to check that all teeth are present, sound and in favourable positions. The absence of third molars will not usually influence treatment unless extraction of second permanent molars is being considered. The absence of any other teeth will, of course, necessitate modifications of the treatment plan.

The Lower Arch

Treatment planning for the lower arch is similar to that for Class II division 1 cases. It is probably best to accept mild crowding. If crowding is marked, extractions, usually of first premolars, are required. For a full discussion of treatment of the crowded lower arch *see* Chapter 11.

The Upper Arch

Treatment planning for the upper arch depends on whether the position of the central incisors (and thus the overbite) is to be accepted or whether it is decided that overbite reduction is necessary. The latter will involve complex fixed appliance treatment.

Where the overbite is to be accepted. If the overbite is not likely to be traumatic and the position of the central incisors is aesthetically acceptable, space is merely required to align the upper teeth. If the crowding is quite mild and the lower arch has been accepted without extractions, distal movement of the upper buccal segments may provide sufficient space. Should upper third molars be present and crowded, the extraction of upper second permanent molars will make this treatment simpler. The appliances used have been described in Chapter 9. Following establishment of a correct intercuspation with the lower arch, the upper canines should be retracted and the lateral incisors aligned. Where crowding in the upper arch is more severe or where there are to be extractions in the lower arch, it will usually be necessary to extract upper 4's,

then 3's retracted.

using an upper removable appliance. Even if it is not intended to reduce the overbite, it is usually worth incorporating an anterior bite plane in the appliance to obviate occlusal interference with canine retraction.

Provided that the upper lateral incisors are not severely rotated, it is usually possible to obtain satisfactory alignment with a labial bow or buccal arms on a removable appliance.

If the upper lateral incisors have to be derotated, it may be necessary to use a simple fixed appliance because this movement is not readily undertaken with a removable appliance.

Where the overbite is to be reduced. If the overbite in a Class II division 2 case is to be reduced and remain stable, it is essential at the same time to reduce the inter-incisor angle. If this is achieved by labial movement of the incisor crowns they may not remain stable but, on removal of the retainers, may relapse lingually into a position of muscle balance. This means that the inter-incisor angle will be increased again and the overbite will relapse.

Stability

Lateral Incisor Alignment

There is a very strong tendency for the lateral incisors to return part of the way towards their original position. This is particularly true if they were rotated. Where possible the position of these teeth should be overcorrected during treatment. Some authorities recommend prolonged retention but it is not yet clear whether retention beyond 6 months does improve stability or whether it merely postpones the relapse. As mentioned in Chapter 7, pericision is sometimes performed on teeth which have been derotated by orthodontic means. There is some evidence that this reduces, even if it does not eliminate, relapse of rotations.

treatment. Some authorities recommend prolonged retention but it is not yet clear whether retention beyond 6 months does improve stability or whether it merely postpones the relapse. As mentioned in Chapter 7, pericision is sometimes performed on teeth which have been derotated by orthodontic means. There is some evidence that this reduces, even if it does not eliminate, relapse of rotations.

Overbites

As discussed under treatment, relapse of overbite reduction will occur unless the inter-incisor angle has been reduced by palatal movement of the incisor apices. It is sometimes suggested that, in Class II division 2 cases, proclination of upper and lower incisors (out of muscle balance) followed by permanent retention should be undertaken. The disadvantages of permanent retainers should not be overlooked: removable retainers will encourage food stagnation and plaque formation with consequent deterioration of the patient's oral health, and if they are left out even for a few weeks, relapse will occur; fixed retainers are complex to make and expensive for the patient and need to be supervised very carefully.

Chapter 16

Class III Malocclusions

OCCLUSAL FEATURES

According to Angle's classification, the lower arch should be at least one-half cusp width too far forward relative to the upper arch. Provided there is a Class III incisor relationship, milder degrees of prenormality are often included in this group of Class III malocclusions (*see Fig.* 6.4).

Labial Segments

The upper incisors are often crowded and they are usually proclined. The lower incisors may be slightly crowded but they are often spaced. Frequently the lower incisors are retroclined. Thus in many cases, the inclination of the incisors compensates to some extent for the sagittal arch malrelationship.

There is a Class III incisor relationship: the lower incisor edges lie anterior to the cingulum plateau of the upper incisors. The lower incisors may lie anterior to the uppers so that there is a reverse overjet (*see Fig.* 6.4). The overbite varies considerably between cases. If there is incisor contact, the overbite will be reduced. Frequently if the anterior intermaxillary height is increased (and there is a large Frankfort mandibular planes angle), there will be an anterior open bite (*see Fig.* 12.1). Occasionally when there is a reverse overjet and the anterior intermaxillary height is low, the overbite is deep.

Buccal Segments

Frequently the upper arch is short so that the buccal segments are crowded: the canines may be mesially inclined and the first permanent molars are distally inclined. In the developing occlusion, second and third molars may be stacked (*see Fig.* 11.1). Where there has been early loss of deciduous molar teeth space loss is rapid in the crowded upper arch. Often the lower arch is long and there may even be spacing.

In the vertical plane, if there is an anterior open bite, this may extend into the buccal segments, and in the most severe cases only the last erupted molars meet in occlusion. Not infrequently, there is a crossbite in the buccal segments. This may be unilateral or bilateral. A unilateral crossbite is usually associated with lateral displacement of the mandible to obtain maximal intercuspation (*see* Chapter 4).

Crossbites in Class III (*see Fig.* 12.1) arise in part because the upper arch is narrow relative to the lower and in part because, with the Class III occlusal relationship, a wider part of the lower arch opposes a given part of the upper.

SKELETAL RELATIONSHIP

The skeletal pattern is the most important factor in producing a Class III malocclusion.

Antero-posterior

Usually there is a Class III skeletal pattern (*Fig.* 16.1). The more adverse the skeletal pattern, the more severe the Class III malocclusion is likely to be and the less amenable to treatment except by surgery.

Although attention is often focused on a large mandible, it must be remembered that a Class III skeletal pattern

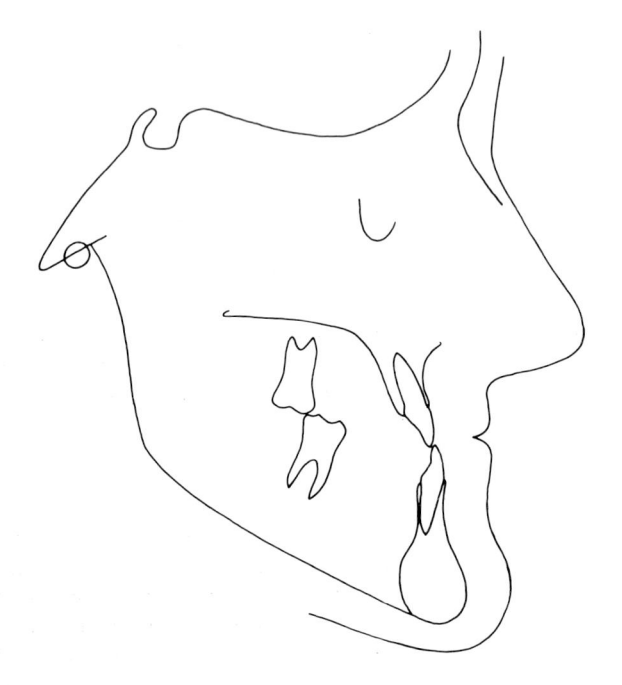

Fig. 16.1. A Class III malocclusion associated with a Class III skeletal pattern.

is frequently also associated with a short retrognathic maxilla and a forward position of the glenoid fossae on the skull base so that the mandible is more anteriorly positioned than usual. Rarely is the skeletal malrelationship due to a single anomalous factor. More commonly it is a combination of factors (mandible, maxilla and cranial base) which, although each is within the normal range, combine to produce a Class III skeletal pattern.

Although the majority of Class III malocclusions are associated with a Class III skeletal pattern, it is possible to have a Class III malocclusion with a Class I skeletal pattern. In these cases the inclination of the teeth or their positions on the skeletal base are responsible for the antero-posterior arch malrelationship.

Vertical

Frequently the anterior height of the intermaxillary space is high. The Frankfort mandibular planes angle is correspondingly high. This is associated with a reduced overbite or anterior open bite. However, is some cases the Frankfort mandibular planes angle is average or even low and the overbite may be normal in amount or deep (with the lower incisors lying anterior to the uppers).

Transverse

In many, but not in all cases, the maxillary base is narrow and the mandibular base wide. The resulting transverse discrepancy is aggravated by the forward position of the mandible relative to the maxilla: as in the case of the dental arches, the skeletal bases diverge posteriorly so that when the lower base is in a forward position, a wider part lies below a given part of the maxilla. In many cases, the transverse discrepancy is compensated for by a buccal inclination of the upper teeth and a lingual inclination of the lower teeth. However, if this is not sufficient there will be a crossbite.

Note: Some authors divide patients with Class III malocclusions into two groups according to their facial pattern. Group 1 has a small, narrow maxilla and a mandible of normal length but with a large gonial angle so that the Frankfort mandibular planes angle is increased. In group 2 the Class III skeletal pattern is due to the large mandible rather than the short maxilla. The Frankfort mandibular planes angle is average or low. Although patients corresponding to these types are found, the majority of Class III cases have features of both groups and so this allocation of patients to groups is not satisfactory. It does, however, draw attention to the wide range of facial patterns which may be associated with Class III malocclusions.

MANDIBULAR POSITIONS AND PATHS OF CLOSURE

Usually there is a simple hinge closure from rest to occlusion. In a number of cases with a mild Class III incisor relationship and a normal or increased overbite, when the mandible is in centric relation, the incisors would meet edge-to-edge (with the posterior teeth out of occlusion) but, in order to obtain a position of maximal occlusion, there is a forward displacement of the mandible which exaggerates the severity of the occlusal and skeletal base malrelationship. A few of these cases may also overclose.

Where there is a unilateral crossbite with the teeth in occlusion there will usually be an associated lateral displacement of the mandible on closure. Patients with occlusal disharmonies and mandibular displacements of the types described above are liable to suffer from muscle pain and so the occlusion should be corrected as early as possible. However, where the maxillary base is narrow and the inclination of the teeth already compensates for this to some extent, simple arch expansion may not be stable.

SOFT TISSUES

Where the anterior intermaxillary height is large the lips are frequently incompetent. These cases often have a skeletal anterior open bite, and during swallowing there will be an adaptive variation of swallowing behaviour with the tongue coming forwards into the gap between the incisors.

ORAL HEALTH

Mandibular displacements due to occlusal disharmonies may be associated with muscle pain. Where there is a premature contact in the incisor region there may be gingival recession around one or more lower incisors, but this is more common in Class I cases with a single instanding upper central incisor. Although in cases where there is an anterior open bite, periodontal changes might be expected around the non-functional teeth (those out of occlusion) no characteristic problems are found.

TREATMENT

The objectives of treatment may include: (1) relief of crowding and alignment of the teeth; (2) correction of the incisor relationship; (3) elimination of a unilateral crossbite.

Generally, the more severe incisor malrelationships are beyond the range of orthodontic treatment, as discussed below.

Treatment Planning

The following discussion is based on the premiss that all permanent teeth except for third molars are present, sound and in favourable positions.

The Lower Arch

The lower arch is often regular or even spaced in which case no treatment is indicated unless an attempt is to be made to retract the lower labial segment. This will be successful only if the lower incisors are proclined and if there will be an overbite at the end of treatment. Fixed appliances are required for treatment of this sort.

If the lower arch is crowded, extraction of lower first premolars should be considered, even if this will provide too much space. The most labially crowded lower incisors will drop back into the line of the arch.

If active retroclination of lower incisors is to be undertaken, then space in the lower premolar region will be required anyway.

The Upper Arch

Relief of crowding. Frequently the upper arch is crowded and extractions are required for its relief.

If the upper permanent canines are mesially inclined and the first permanent molars are distally inclined, the extraction of upper premolars, usually first premolars, is called for. Sometimes due to narrowness of the upper arch, the canines are distally inclined and lie over the lateral incisors. In these circumstances it may be more appropriate to extract the lateral incisors if they are palatally displaced or the canines if the lateral incisors are in the line of the arch and there are good approximal contacts with the first premolars. However, should premolars still be the teeth of choice for extraction despite the distal inclination of the canines, fixed appliances will be required.

Overjet. If there is a positive but reduced overjet or if the incisors meet edge to edge when the teeth are in maximal occlusion, this should be accepted. When there is a reverse overjet the decison must be made whether it is feasible to correct it. The following factors should be taken into account:

1. Can the patient obtain an edge-to-edge occlusion of the incisors by retracting the mandible ? If not, the prognosis for correction of the reverse overjet is poor.

2. Would there be an overbite following correction of the reverse overjet? If not, correction of the overjet will not be stable. Even if there is an overbite before treatment, it must be recognized that this will be reduced as the

incisors are tipped forwards by a removable appliance. Sometimes it will be found that only the central incisors have an overbite. In this case, particularly if the lateral incisors were initially crowded further palatally than the central incisors, the lateral incisors will usually relapse into lingual occlusion following treatment.

3. Are the upper incisors already proclined? If they are, it may not be possible to tip them further forwards without prejudicing their periodontal health: if the upper incisors are excessively proclined, the occlusion of the lower incisors will load them transversly rather than axially and this may promote periodontal breakdown and wandering of the teeth.

Unless the Class III skeletal pattern is very mild, orthodontic treatment to correct the sagittal arch malrelationship is not usually possible. Quite apart from this, it is frequently the mandibular prominence rather than the reverse overjet which is of concern to the patient. Surgical treatment to correct the skeletal pattern may be indicated in these cases (Chapter 19).

Overbite. If there is a skeletal open bite it cannot be corrected by orthodontic means. Extrusion of the teeth by fixed appliances is possible but may not be stable. In addition, extrusion of incisors in cases of skeletal open bite is not usually accompanied by corresponding growth in height of the alveolar bone and so the ratio of crown length to root length of the tooth is adversely increased. A mild degree of anterior open bite is not usually a matter of concern to the patient, although it may prevent the stable correction of a reverse overjet. The only treatment for a severe skeletal open bite is surgical, although this is rarely justified unless surgical correction of the Class III skeletal pattern is to be undertaken at the same time.

Crossbite. Where there is a unilateral crossbite with lateral displacement of the mandible on closure, expansion of the upper arch to eliminate the crossbite may be successful. A bilateral crossbite should be accepted. The treatment of crossbites is discussed at length in Chapter 12.

Stability

Stability of overjet correction depends in the short term on an adequate overbite and in the long term on facial growth. The greater part of orthodontic treatment is undertaken in the growing patient. On average, the mandible grows downwards and forwards slightly faster than the maxilla. In Class III patients this is an adverse growth trend and may result both in a worsening (or relapse) of the overjet and a reduction in overbite. In some patients the Class III skeletal pattern will become markedly more severe after treatment and in these cases relapse is inevitable. In other patients the facial proportions change little during the later stages of growth and no adverse occlusal changes should result. In Class III, more than other types of malocclusion, long term stability depends on a favourable growth pattern.

Chapter 17

Fixed Appliances

Fixed appliances are powerful and complex mechanisms and their unskilled use may lead to extensive and rapid unwanted tooth movements. The dental practitioner without special training should not attempt to use fixed appliances. However, he may need to refer patients requiring fixed appliance treatment to an orthodontic specialist. Thus he should have some knowledge of their scope and action.

Definition. A fixed appliance is an orthodontic device where attachments are fixed to the teeth and forces applied by arch wires or auxiliaries through these attachments. This allows precise control over the nature and direction of the forces applied.

COMPONENTS OF FIXED APPLIANCES

Attachments

The attachments (brackets, tubes, etc.) are peculiar to each fixed appliance technique. Their function is to allow a controlled force (or couple of forces) to be applied to the tooth (*Fig.* 17.1). The attachments are fixed to the teeth either by means of etch-retained composite resins (*Fig.* 17.2), or by being welded to stainless steel bands which are then cemented to the teeth (*Fig.* 17.3). Bands may be purchased in a variety of stock sizes or may be made up from stainless steel tape. Directly bonded attachments are less conspicuous than bands, but during bonding, the tooth must be kept absolutely dry. They are used on

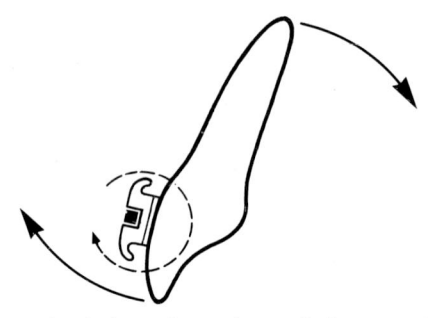

Fig. 17.1. A mechanical couple can be applied to a tooth with a fixed appliance. This means that precise control over root movement is possible.

anterior teeth while molars, particularly if extra-oral traction is to be applied, are usually banded.

Archwires

Depending on the technique, round or rectangular archwires may be used and are fixed to the brackets by soft wire ligatures, plastic rings or pins. The archwire may be active (the archwire is deflected on tying in to the attachments so that forces are applied to the teeth), or passive (the archwire is not deflected but forces are applied by auxiliary springs or elastics). Active archwires often have loops bent into them (*Fig.* 17.3*a*) to increase their flexibility at sites of irregularity or where spaces have to be opened or closed.

Auxiliaries

Forces may be applied to the teeth by auxiliary springs or elastics. Latex elastics are used for transmitting forces between the arches (intermaxillary traction) as well as within the one arch (intramaxillary traction).

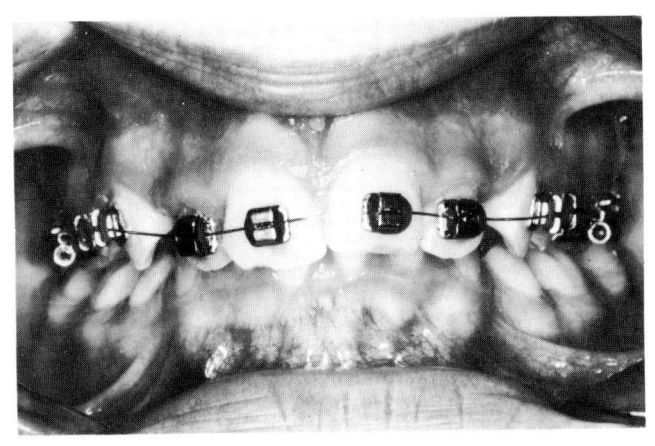

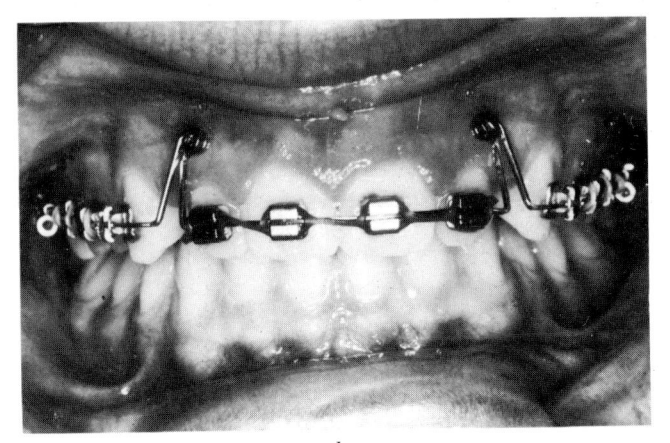

Fig. 17.2. An edgewise appliance with directly bonded attachments. *a*, A thin round wire archwire is used to obtain initial alignment of the teeth and, *b*, precise control of tooth positions is achieved by the use of rectangular archwires. The loops in this archwire are active components to retract the incisors.

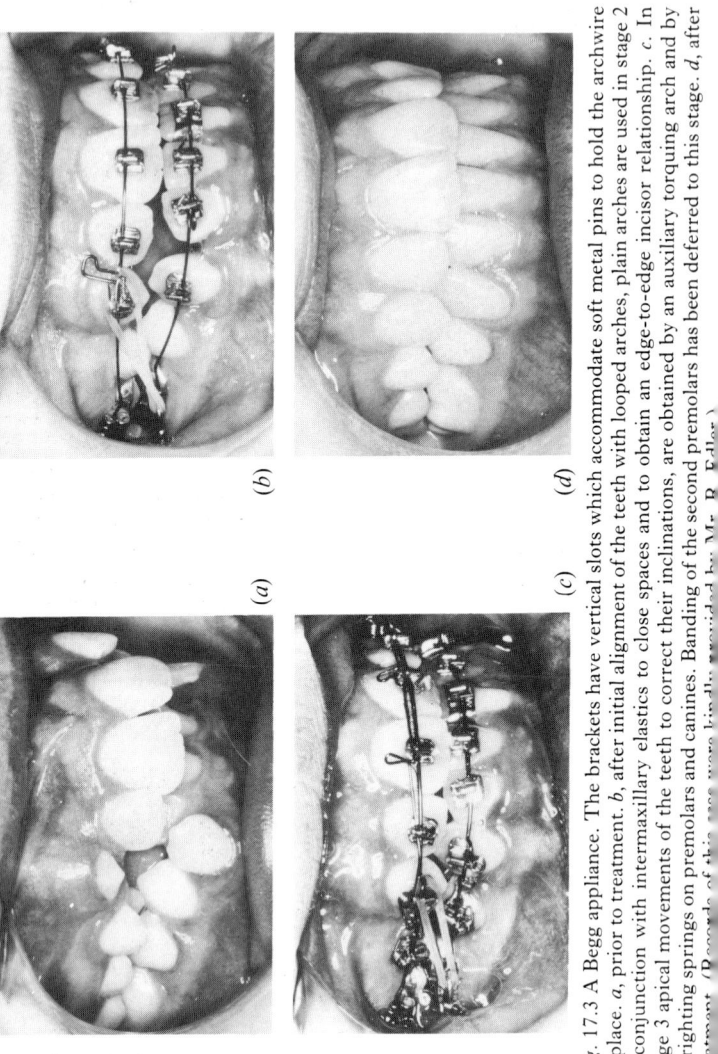

Fig. 17.3 A Begg appliance. The brackets have vertical slots which accommodate soft metal pins to hold the archwire in place. *a*, prior to treatment. *b*, after initial alignment of the teeth with looped arches, plain arches are used in stage 2 in conjunction with intermaxillary elastics to close spaces and to obtain an edge-to-edge incisor relationship. *c*, In stage 3 apical movements of the teeth to correct their inclinations, are obtained by an auxiliary torquing arch and by uprighting springs on premolars and canines. Banding of the second premolars has been deferred to this stage. *d*, after

ADVANTAGES AND DISADVANTAGES OF FIXED COMPARED WITH REMOVABLE APPLIANCES

Fixed	*Removable*
1. Precise control over force distribution to individual teeth means that rotation and controlled root movement are possible.	Single point application of forces means that only tipping movements are readily produced.
2. Multiple tooth movements can be performed simultaneously.	Usually only a few teeth should be moved at any one time.
3. Complex to make and use so special training is needed.	Comparatively simple and should be within the scope of the dental practitioner for carefully selected cases.
4. Chairside time is comparatively long.	Chairside time is short but laboratory time greater than for fixed appliances.
5. Components are costly.	Components are inexpensive.
6. Oral hygiene is made more difficult.	As the appliance is removable the problems of oral hygiene should not be increased.

LIMITATIONS OF FIXED APPLIANCES

It should be recognized that many of the limitations of removable appliance treatment apply equally to fixed appliances.

1. Patient cooperation is required, even although the appliance is fixed. The uncooperative patient will not maintain an adequate standard of oral hygiene, will not wear intra-oral elastics or headgear as directed and may intentionally or carelessly damage his appliances. Thus fixed appliance treatment is not appropriate for the uncooperative child who will not wear removable appliances.

2. The rate of tooth movement is limited by the biological response of the supporting tissues. This is the same, regardless of the type of appliance used.

3. Treatment effects are limited to the teeth and alveolar structures. While it is possible by controlled tooth movement with fixed appliances to obtain good occlusion even where the skeletal relationship is unfavourable, the improvement in the patient's facial appearance may not match the improvement in occlusion. Where the skeletal pattern is very adverse, it is not possible to obtain a good occlusion, even with fixed appliances.

4. Stability of treatment with fixed appliances depends on exactly the same factors as with removable appliances: the position of balance depends on the harmonious interaction between skeletal relationship, soft tissue pattern and interdental forces.

FIXED APPLIANCE TECHNIQUES

Multiband techniques

A variety of techniques is available in which attachments are fitted to most or all of the teeth. Archwires are designed so that controlled tooth movement in any plane of space is possible. The most widely known are the Edgewise and the Begg techniques.

Edgewise technique

Attachments with rectangular slots are used (*Fig.* 17.2). Light round arches may be fitted for initial alignment but for controlled tooth movement in all planes of space rectangular archwires are used. The Edgewise technique was introduced by Angle, and at the present time a number of variations are in use.

Begg technique

In contrast with the Edgewise technique, the attachments have simple vertical slots which allow free tipping of the teeth (*Fig.* 17.3). Round archwires are used and controlled root movement in any direction is obtained by the use of auxiliary springs.

FIXED–REMOVABLE APPLIANCES

Sometimes it is useful to be able to use fixed attachments in association with a removable appliance. Particularly where retention is liable to be poor and it is desirable to use extra-oral traction, bands may be cemented to upper molars to carry a facebow (*Fig.* 17.4). This can be used alone to retract the upper molars, or to reinforce anchorage in conjunction with a removable appliance. In that case modified clasps to fit over the tubes on the molar

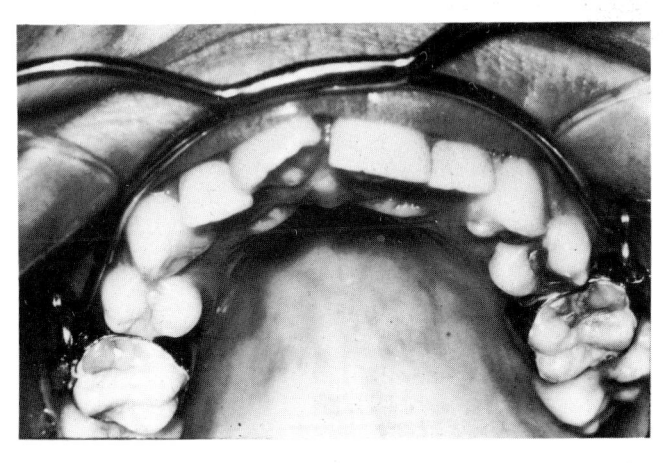

Fig. 17.4. Bands cemented to first permanent molars carry tubes into which the ends of the facebow can be slipped. This, together with the headgear, is worn at nights or as prescribed.

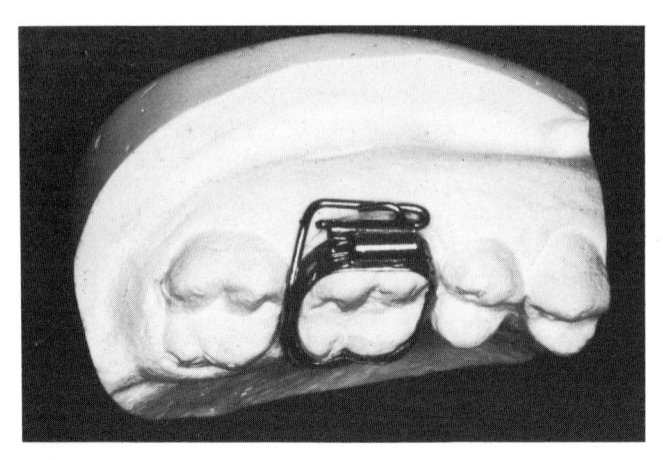

Fig. 17.5. A modified molar clasp for an upper removable appliance to be worn in conjunction with the bands on the molars.

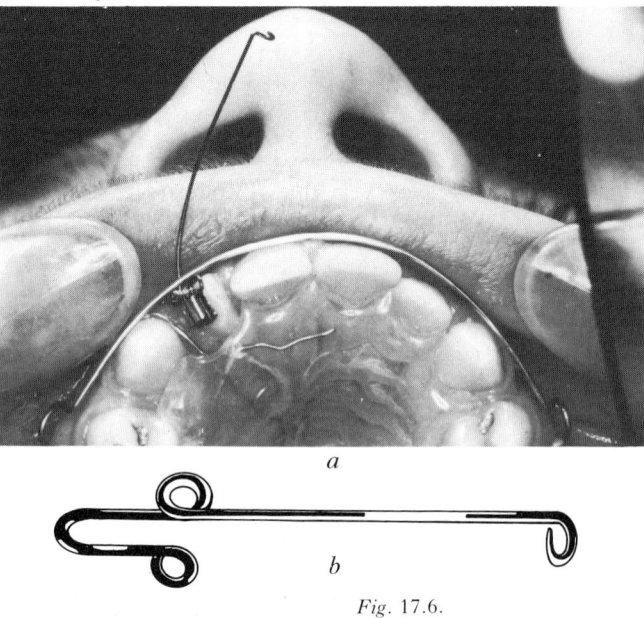

Fig. 17.6.

bands, are used on the appliance (*Fig.* 17.5). Where one or perhaps two incisors are rotated, a whip and bonded attachment used in conjunction with a removable appliance (*Fig.* 17.6) is effective. Directly bonded attachments are particularly useful in this context as only a small stock needs to be carried and a composite filling material can be used as the adhesive after etching the enamel surface in the usual manner.

Fig. 17.6. *a*, A whip on the upper lateral incisor with a directly bonded edgewise bracket. *b* shows the design of the whip which is made from 0·5 mm wire. It clips over the wings of the bracket and is held in place by a ligature wire twisted through the loops in the wire. The free end of the whip clips over the labial bow and a rotational couple is applied to the tooth. The patient can take out the removable appliance for cleaning.

Chapter 18

Functional Appliances

Functional appliances utilize the forces of the orofacial muscles to move teeth. The fact that they depend on muscle forces in no way implies a special mode of action: they produce their effects as a result of tooth movement brought about by the tissue changes described in Chapter 7. The major effect of functional appliances is on the position of the teeth and alveolar processes. There is still much debate about the possibility of orthopaedic effects, with some evidence that in favourable cases, mandibular condylar growth may be enhanced or redirected. Many functional appliances have been described but only the most important examples from each group will be mentioned. For a detailed account of their construction *see* Adams (1984).

THE ORAL SCREEN

This appliance (*Fig.* 18.1) is a thin shield of acrylic which lies in the buccal sulcus. It is worn at night. In its passive form it transmits the forces of the circumoral musculature uniformly to the teeth. The passive oral screen has been used as a retainer (following upper incisor retraction in Class II division 1 cases) and to discourage thumb sucking.

In its active form it contacts only the upper incisors and stands away from the other teeth so that the muscular forces are concentrated on the upper incisors. The passive screen may be made active by adding a thin layer of cold-cure acrylic to the screen where it contacts the upper incisors. The active oral screen has been used for overjet reduction in cases where there is sufficient incisor spacing

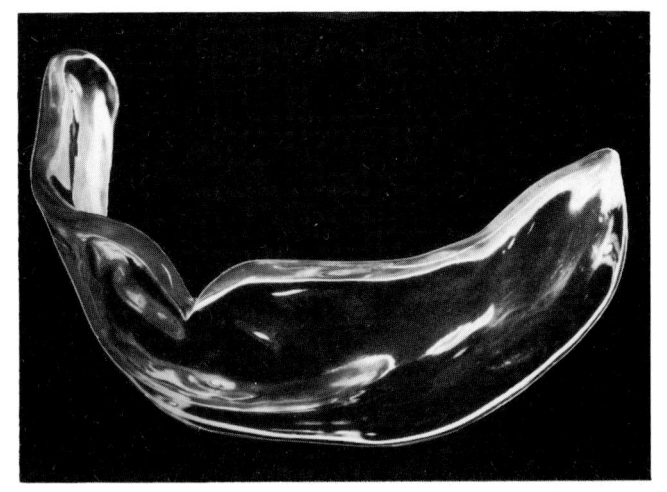

Fig. 18.1. An oral screen.

incomplete so that the lower incisors do not interfere with the upper incisor retraction. It is probably fair to say that the same result can be obtained more quickly and with less inconvenience to the patient by normal removable appliances.

THE ANDRESEN APPLIANCE

This appliance (*Fig.* 18.2) was developed from the monobloc of Robin. It consists of upper and lower appliances sealed together so that the forces of the muscles of mastication can be transmitted between the arches. Although a variety of malocclusions may be treated by the expert, the general use of the Andresen appliance is confined to carefully selected Class II division 1 cases with the following features:

1. The arches must be uncrowded and in regular alignment. It is advantageous if the lower incisors are spaced. The upper molars must not be inclined distally.

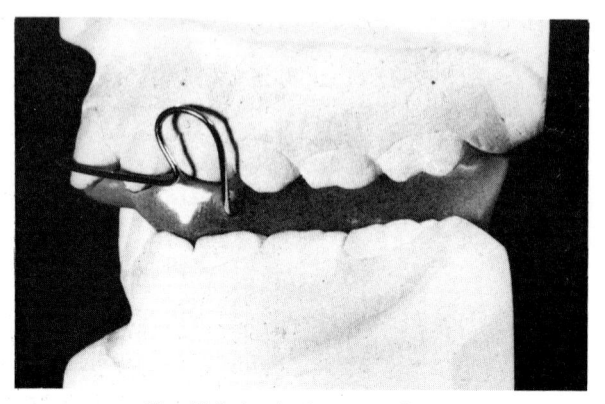

Fig. 18.2. An Andresen appliance.

2. The lower arch should be not more than one-half cusp width distal to the upper.
3. The skeletal pattern should be Class I or mild Class II.
4. There must be no habit posture of the mandible.

For success, the working bite and laboratory procedures must be carried out carefully. The working bite is taken with the mandible symmetrically postured forwards to obtain a Class I buccal segment relationship and opened about 2 mm beyond the freeway space. This means that when the appliance is fitted the mandible is held forwards and the muscles acting on it (in particular the posterior fibres of temporalis) tend to retract it to its normal position. As a result forces are generated which tend to move the upper teeth distally and the lower teeth mesially. This is an example of intermaxillary traction. In order to facilitate tooth movement and allow overbite reduction, channels are trimmed over the occlusal surfaces of the molars and premolars. These channels are directed backwards in the upper arch and forwards in the lower. As a result, the appliance contacts the upper posterior teeth only on their mesiopalatal aspects and the lowers only on their distolingual aspects. This guides their direction of eruption to encourage correction of the occlusion. It is important that, in the construction of the appliance, the acrylic should be carried over the lower incisor tips. The capping acts as a bite plane to permit overbite reduction and is meant to prevent the lower incisors from tipping forwards. However, a major problem with the Andresen appliance is that the lower incisors may be moved labially out of muscle balance and will relapse when treatment is completed.

The patient is instructed to wear the appliance at night and for as many hours as possible each day. With careful case selection good results may be obtained, but the dental practitioner can usually treat these cases more readily by using conventional removable appliances. For example, the mild uncrowded Class II division 1 malocclusion may be treated by using extra-oral traction to retract the upper buccal segments, followed by overjet reduction, without any risk of disturbing the balance of the lower arch.

THE FRÄNKEL APPLIANCE

This is a variety of functional appliance (*Fig.* 18.3). In principle it differs from the Andresen appliance in that its action primarily depends on acrylic shields which are designed to hold the lips and cheeks away from the teeth, so disturbing the muscle balance and producing tooth movement. In Class II cases, the appliance is designed to hold the mandible in a forward position. The appliance is described by Fränkel as a 'function regulator' (FR) and, as its name implies, he believes that it permanently modifies the position and activities of the orofacial muscles and promotes growth at the mandibular condyle. At the present time there is no objective evidence to support these concepts.

Treatment with the Fränkel appliance is usually begun in the early mixed dentition. The appliance is worn part

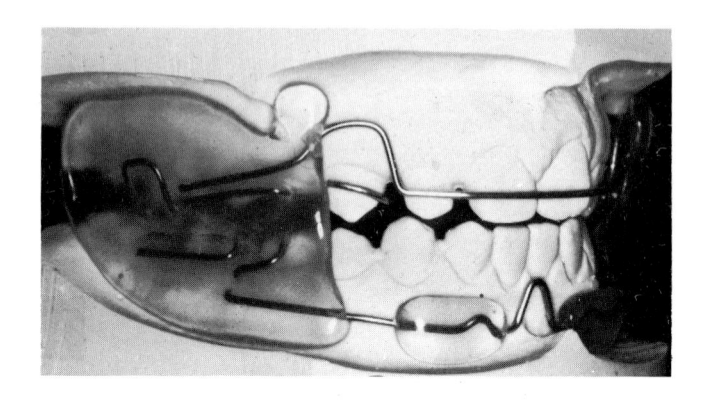

Fig. 18.3. The Fränkel appliance.

time until the patient is accustomed to it, then full time. Although the appropriate design of Fränkel appliance can be used to treat any arch malrelationship, it is used most commonly in Class II division 1 malocclusions. Crowding in Class II cases is not a contraindication to its use as some arch expansion is produced, but clearly the result will not be stable unless the teeth are in a position of muscle balance at the end of treatment.

Reference

Adams C. P. (1984) *The Design and Construction of Removable Orthodontic Appliances,* 5th ed. Bristol, Wright.

Chapter 19

Oral Surgery in Relation to Orthodontics

Surgical techniques are described in detail by Howe (1985).

MINOR ORAL SURGERY

Lower third molars and upper canines are the teeth most frequently misplaced and impacted. Impaction may be due to crowding or to an abnormal developmental position of the tooth germ. An impacted or displaced tooth rarely causes symptoms unless there is an associated pathological lesion (e.g. a cyst) or the mucosa is breached. Before any unerupted tooth is removed, a careful clinical and radiographic assessment must be made.

Maxillary canines

Permanent upper canines develop beneath the orbital border and have a long path of eruption. During eruption they may be deflected, usually palatally. Where an upper permanent canine has not yet erupted in a child over 13 years of age, an investigation is necessary. Not only must the position of the canine tooth be determined precisely, but the following features should be looked for.
 1. Resorption of incisor roots.
 2. Cystic change of the follicle.
 3. Apical dilaceration.
 4. Displacement of related teeth.
 A full orthodontic diagnosis must be made and the

chances of eruption either normally or after surgical exposure must be estimated. Possible lines of treatment are as follows.

Leave Alone

This can be recommended only if the canine is asymptomatic, with no evidence or likelihood of infection, cystic change or resorption of adjacent teeth (e.g. where a horizontal canine is very high within the palate). Regular annual review of these patients is essential.

Surgical Exposures

The following criteria must be fulfilled:

1. The canine is favourably positioned with its apex close to the correct position.

2. The potential path of eruption is not obstructed.

3. Adequate room is available within the dental arch, achieved either orthodontically or by extraction, usually of a first premolar.

A generous exposure of the area of the crown should be accomplished by removing the overlying palatal mucosa. The labial mucoperiosteum should *not* be removed. The crown of the canine must be uncovered to clear the tip of the crown, the cingulum and the maximal mediodistal diameter of the tooth. The buccal plate should be left intact and the root of the tooth must not be touched. Bone in the direction of desired eruption may be removed so long as these two principles are not contravened.

The wound is packed for at least 10 days. An appliance may be required to maintain the space and this will require adjustment as the tooth erupts.

Extraction

This may be indicated where:

1. The tooth is too badly displaced to erupt normally or with orthodontic assistance, and can be removed without undue danger to other teeth.

2. There is pathological change (e.g. cystic change or resorption).

3. There is an intact arch where its absence would not be detrimental.

Transplantation

In carefully selected cases, with no medical contra-indications, it is possible to undertake transplantation, thereby avoiding prosthetic replacement.

Space must be available, and success is more likely where the apex is open. The root should not be handled or bruised by instrumentation. Root filling should not be attempted at the time of transplantation but left, should it prove necessary, until the tooth is firm in its new position. Ankylosis of the tooth and resorption of the root may occur.

Mandibular Third Molars

Impaction is a common problem (*see* p. 122). Orthodontic treatment cannot be considered complete until the wisdom teeth have erupted fully into occlusion or have been extracted.

Early Removal

In carefully selected cases the lower third molars may be removed by lateral trepanation (Burgess et al., 1971) at an early stage under outpatient intubation general anaesthesia, without disturbance to the second molars, their bone or periodontium. Experience has shown that healing is rapid and the incidence of postoperative problems is low. However, this is a technique for the experienced and specifically trained operator. Strict criteria of selection must be applied:

1. A healthy child with a healthy mouth.

2. A full orthodontic assessment and a clear indication that there is little or no chance of the lower third molars erupting into a normal and useful position.
3. The crowns formed, but with root development no more than one-third complete.
4. The tooth completely covered by bone.

Later Removal

If impaction or lack of space cannot be confidently predicted, then the third molar is put on probation. Usually by the late teens, at a stage when just over two-thirds of the root formation is complete, a decision should be made concerning its removal. Surgically this is the optimal time for the late removal of wisdom teeth, and is before any serious damage has resulted to the adjacent teeth or periodontium.

Supernumerary Teeth

The orthodontic aspects have been discussed in Chapter 10. A supernumerary tooth should be removed provided that this will not endanger the vitality of the other teeth. However, if the supernumerary is symptomless, and very deeply buried it may be better to leave it in situ. Before surgery is undertaken, accurate localization is absolutely essential (*see* p. 112).

In the majority of cases, remembering the age of patient and the difficulty of access, these teeth are best removed under intubation general anaesthesia. The surgical approach depends upon their position and the same principles apply as with removal of unerupted canine teeth. It must be stressed that a minimum of bone should be removed to gain access to the supernumerary and great care taken not to interfere with the permanent teeth. Exposure of the normal incisors and interference with their follicles should be avoided as this may lead to the formation of scar tissue, which in itself will impede eruption and so necessitate a later operation to uncover the incisor.

Unerupted Incisor Teeth

These occasionally require surgical exposure to facilitate their eruption. The criteria are similar to the surgical exposure of canine teeth.

Although the teeth may be palpated buccally above the reflection of the mucous membrane, the temptation to make an incision here must be resisted. The gum should be incised on the alveolar ridge, palatal to the buried tooth. The flap is reflected and mobilized upwards and forwards so that it can be apically repositioned to show the incisal edge. By this means the depth of the labial sulcus is maintained and a sound gingival margin is obtained.

The incisal edge, cingulum and maximal mesiodistal diameter of the tooth must be exposed by removing bone prior to repositioning of the flap.

Fraenectomy

The operation is designed to remove the fraenum and the fibrous tissue lying in the intermaxillary suture between the roots of the central incisor teeth. A fraenectomy may be done under local anaesthesia with a co-operative child, but otherwise requires general anaesthesia as the operation needs to be done carefully and thoroughly. The fraenal band is removed as for fraenoplasty (*see* Howe, 1985), but with the excision of tissue down to bone as it extends between the central incisors to the incisive papilla. Then, the intermaxillary suture is cleared of fibrous tissue up to at least the level of the apices of the incisors. The mucosa of the lip is undermined and the edges are closed by simple sutures. Healing is usually rapid, the sutures being removed after 7 days.

DENTO-ALVEOLAR SURGERY

Occasionally where a patient is unsuitable for or is unwilling to undergo orthodontic treatment, a labial segment malrelationship may be corrected by dento-alveolar surgery. A block of teeth and alveolar bone (*Fig.* 19.1) together with sufficient soft tissue to maintain a blood supply is surgically repositioned. Where there is a marked dental base malrelationship, this may be corrected at the same time by more major jaw surgery (*see* p. 184).

It must be recognized that the stability of surgically repositioned teeth depends on the same factors as orthodontic treatment. Dento-alveolar surgery is usually limited to cases where the teeth are well aligned.

The surgical principles may be illustrated by the lower labial set-back mandibular ostectomy. The procedure is entirely intra-oral.

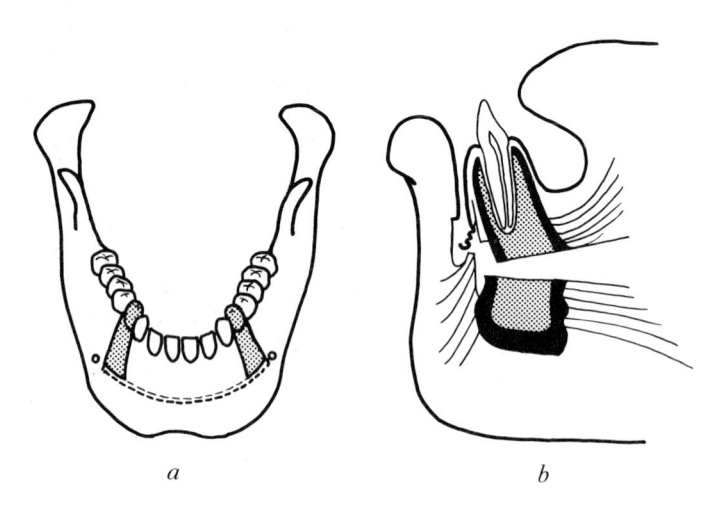

Fig. 19.1. *a*, The bone cuts for a lower labial set-back. *b*, Showing the soft tissue incision (labially) and the lingual pedicle through which the blood supply is maintained.

Lower Labial Set-back Mandibular Ostectomy (*Fig.* 19.1)

This may be used to correct a Class III incisor relationship with a moderate reverse overjet. If the Class III skeletal pattern is severe, more major jaw surgery is required.

Careful preoperative planning with a full orthodontic assessment is essential. In addition to the standard orthodontic radiographs, good periapical views are required to show the position of the teeth and mental foramina so that the ostectomy cuts can be planned. Articulated plaster models are sectioned to simulate the operation and to determine the site and size of bone cuts.

The operation is performed under inpatient general anaesthesia. It is not a major procedure and the period in hospital is only 3–4 days. In order to create space for the distal positioning of the segment of alveolus bearing the lower labial segment, lower first premolars are usually extracted, although occasionally pre-existing gaps can be used. The vertical cuts are made in front of the mental foramina and only the incisive branches of the inferior dental nerves are divided. If the mental nerve should be in the line of the osteotomy cut it can be repositioned surgically. A subapical horizontal cut completes the ostectomy. The blood supply is via the lingual pedicle which is maintained intact.

Segmental cap splints with preplanned locking bars fix the segments accurately into position for 6 weeks. No intermaxillary fixation is required, thereby avoiding the attendant airway and feeding problems. After taking off the cap splints a removable acrylic retention plate is worn for 3–6 months, while the bony union consolidates.

The ostectomy reduces the tongue space. Careful follow-up is required. If any relapse occurs, a reduction in tongue size by an anterior wedge resection must be considered. However, this is required only in a minority of cases.

The basic procedure is capable of considerable variation and the more common will be mentioned.

Lower Labial Set-down

This may be used to reduce an excessive overbite to allow distal movement of the upper labial segment.

Lower Labial Set-up (Köle Procedure)

This is used to close an open bite which is confined to the anterior part of the dental arches. (If the maxillary anterior segment is also at fault, this may have to be repositioned at the same time by a Wassmund-type procedure.) The lower labial segment is elevated and repositioned to close the anterior open bite. The subapical space thus formed is closed by a slice of bone taken from the lower border of the mandible in the region of the chin.

Anterior Maxillary Ostectomy (Wassmund Procedure)

Where there is a *true* maxillary protrusion with a relatively normal mandibular position, the premaxillary segment carrying the upper incisors and canine teeth may be set back after space has been provided distally by bone removal. Usually the upper first premolars have to be extracted.

Prior to surgery the inclination of the incisors and the inter-canine width may be corrected orthodontically so that the segment can be moved straight back. Rotation of the segment forms a palatal step and gives poor bony contact. A deep over-bite should be corrected either by orthodontic treatment before surgery or by a lower labial set-down.

MAJOR ORTHODONTIC SURGERY

Where there is a severe Class II or Class III skeletal pattern, orthodontic treatment to correct the associated malocclusion may not be possible. Quite apart from this, correction of the tooth position will not materially improve the facial appearance of these patients. Surgery may be used to modify or correct the skeletal disproportion.

Treatment Planning

Details of the radiographs, study models and photographs used in preoperative planning are not given. However, two problems must be defined:

1. Which part of the facial skeleton is at fault? A Class III skeletal pattern, for example, may result from an unduly prognathic mandible or from a retrognathic maxilla. Severe deformities arise when both conditions are present to a marked degree.

2. Would a change in dental base relationship lead to a stable and functional correction of the malocclusion? Correction of the skeletal relationship usually leads to an improvement both in appearance and in occlusion. Where a compromise between aesthetics and function is necessary, priority should be given to obtaining a good functional occlusion.

Stability of surgical repositioning of the jaws may be influenced by:

1. Continued growth. Surgical correction of skeletal abnormalities in growing children may not be stable if the growth pattern is adverse. For this reason, jaw surgery is best done when growth is complete, but dento-alveolar surgery may be undertaken at an earlier age.

2. Soft Tissue Environment. (*a*) *Investing Soft Tissue*: Where there is insufficient soft tissue within which to move the facial bones, relapse will occur into a position of equilibrium. (*b*) *Muscle*: When a bone is repositioned, the main muscle groups must be allowed to take up a position where their original lengths and lines of action remain unaltered. If this is not done, then muscle action will tend to cause a relapse.

Mandibular Prognathism

This is the commonest type of facial disproportion to be corrected surgically. Apart from the aesthetic problem, there is usually a severe malocclusion with disruption of masticatory function.

In certain cases the appearance of mandibular prognathism is secondary to a maxillary retrognathism, but unless this is severe an acceptable result may be obtained by mandibular surgery alone.

Numerous techniques to correct mandibular prognathism are described in standard texts. A number of these procedures (such as a body ostectomy) do have a place in treating individual cases, but only two are now generally accepted: these are the Sagittal Splitting Technique of Obwegeser (*Fig.* 19.2) and the Vertical Subsigmoid Osteotomy.

The Obwegeser technique will be described in more detail as it exemplifies the basic principles. It has greater flexibility and may also be used for correction of mandibular retrognathism.

However, these techniques have in common the following advantages:

1. The entire horizontal body of the mandible is moved back in relation to an undisplaced ascending ramus. Thus

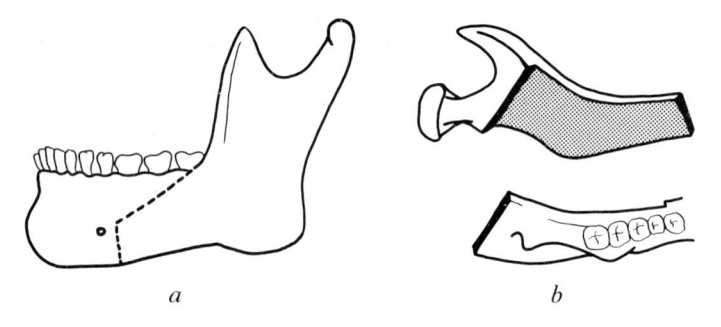

Fig. 19.2. *a*, The lateral bone cuts for a sagittal split osteotomy. *b*, An 'exploded' view to show the bone cuts following the split.

the mandibular tongue attachments and the floor of the mouth are moved backwards, without any diminution of the tongue space within the dental arch.

2. There is no interference with the dental arch.

3. The surgical approach, which is essentially subperiosteal, ensures that the masseter and medial pterygoid muscles are completely freed from their lower attachments. This is taken further by dividing any deep fascia and fibrous connection between them, i.e. the 'pterygomasseteric sling'. This allows the muscles to reattach to the bone, without tension, after a change in the bony position.

The vertical subsigmoid osteotomy is usually done via external skin incisions, and therefore carries the disadvantage of facial scarring and possible facial nerve damage.

Mandibular Osteotomy (Fig. 19.2)

The sagittal split mandibular osteotomy was first described by Obwegeser in 1957, and since that time, with certain modifications, it has become a standard procedure for the correction of mandibular prognathism, retrognathism and of certain types of anterior open bite.

The operation, which is conducted subperiosteally in the region of the ascending ramus and posterior part of the body of mandible, consists of splitting the bone in the sagittal plane between medial and lateral cortical plates, thereby allowing the fragments to slide one upon the other. The body of the mandible can now be brought forwards or set backwards (with a degree of vertical rotation if required) to the preplanned position.

The sagittal split provides a broad area of bony contact, thereby ensuring rapid union. Intermaxillary fixation is held usually for a least 6 weeks.

Mandibular Retrognathism

Patients referred for surgical correction of a mandibular retrognathism have a severe skeletal malrelationship.

Commonly there is a traumatic incisor relationship with the lower incisors biting on to the palatal gingivae. In Class II division 2 malocclusions the lower labial gingivae may be damaged by the retroclined upper incisors. Many adult patients seek help, not for aesthetic but for functional reasons.

It is not possible in the space available to go into details of the management of these interesting and often difficult cases. However, at the risk of over-simplification it can be stated that the essential procedure in the majority of these cases is to lengthen the mandible. This is done by a sagittal splitting technique (Obwegeser) with the advancement of the anterior fragment.

Before this is undertaken preparatory orthodontic treatment may be needed:

1. The incisor inclination is corrected to as near normal as possible. In Class II division 1 cases the upper incisors are retroclined and the interdental spaces closed. Class II division 2 patients will have their incisor relationship converted to the division 1 type and are then treated surgically as such.

2. The intercanine and interpremolar width must be sufficient to receive the repositioned lower dental arch.

3. The excessive overbite must be reduced. In mild cases this may be done by depressing the lower incisors orthodontically. Where the overbite is extreme it will be corrected by a lower labial segment set-down 3–4 weeks prior to the mandibular osteotomy.

In certain patients, where there is a very low Frankfort mandibular plane angle and a reduction in the lower facial height, a modification of this procedure may be used. The mandible is advanced, but with a rotation of the chin downwards to open the gonial angle, decrease the overbite and correct the incisor relationship. A lateral open bite in the premolar region is produced but in the young adult this will close by eruption of the teeth.

References

Burgess P. T., Houston W. J. B. and Howe G. L. (1971) *Dent. Practit.* **22**, 69–72.

Howe G. L. (1985) *Minor Oral Surgery*, 3rd ed. Bristol, Wright.

Chapter 20

Clefts of the Lip and Palate

The prevalence of clefts of the lip and palate varies between racial groups but in Caucasians it is about 1 in 1000.

AETIOLOGY

There is often a history of clefts of lip and palate within a family but the mode of inheritance is not simple. Many environmental insults to the embryo can produce clefts in animals but whether these are of any significance in human populations is uncertain.

Embryologically, the palate can be divided into the primary palate, which develops from fusion of the facial processes and gives rise to the upper lip and palate anterior to the incisive foramen; and the secondary palate, which arises from fusion of the palatal processes and gives rise to the hard palate posterior to the incisive foramen, and to the soft palate. It is thought that clefts of the primary palate result from failure of mesenchymal consolidation whereas clefts of the secondary palate may arise if the palatal processes fail to come into contact. Details of the embryology are available in the standard texts (e.g. Ross and Johnston).

CLASSIFICATION

Many classifications of clefts of lip and palate have been proposed but none is entirely satisfactory. For the individual patient it is probably most convenient just to describe the defect. However, for purposes of description it is useful to divide clefts in three groups:

1. Clefts of the primary palate: may involve only the lip or the lip and alveolar process as far back as the incisive foramen (*Fig.* 20.1*a*).

2. Clefts of the secondary palate: may involve the soft palate only or the soft palate and hard palate as far forwards as the incisive foramen (*Fig.* 20.1*d*).

3. Clefts involving both the primary and secondary palate (*Fig.* 20.1*b* and *c*).

Clefts of the Primary Palate (*Fig.* 20.1*a*)

The deformity varies from notching of the lip to a complete lip cleft with alveolar involvement. The orthodontic and dental problems are local ones superimposed on the normal range of malocclusions. The alveolar cleft is in the lateral incisor area with the result that anomalies of this tooth are often seen: it may be absent or poorly developed and/or malpositioned; or there may be dichotomy of the lateral incisor with one small peg-shaped tooth on either side of the cleft line. The central incisor on the side of the cleft is often rotated and hypoplastic.

Normally the arch form is good. Conventional orthodontic treatment may be indicated and a fixed or removable prosthesis may be required to replace missing or malformed teeth in the region of the cleft.

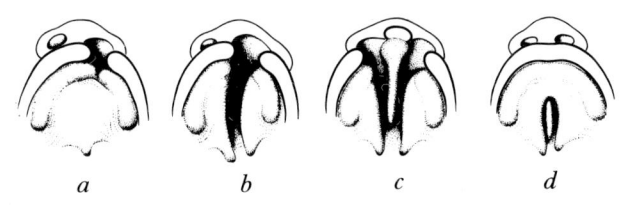

Fig. 20.1. Clefts of the lip and palate. *a*, Cleft of the primary palate (lip and alveolar process). *b*, A unilateral complete cleft of the lip and palate. *c*, A bilateral complete cleft of the lip and palate. *d*, A cleft of the secondary palate.

Clefts of the Secondary Palate (*Fig.* 20.1*d*)

These vary from a submucous cleft of the soft palate to a complete cleft of the soft and hard palate as far forward as the incisive canal.

A cleft of the soft palate alone causes little skeletal disturbance but may be associated with micrognathia and glossoptosis (the Pierre Robin syndrome). In the latter group, there may be respiratory and feeding problems during the first few weeks after birth. Good nursing is usually all that is required but special cradles in which the baby is suspended face down, to keep the tongue forwards, have been described.

Where the hard palate has been repaired, the upper arch is often narrow with the result that some crowding and a crossbite (uni- or bilateral) may be present. Orthodontic alignment of teeth follows conventional lines, but midface growth is unpredictable and a Class III relationship may develop by the time the patient reaches maturity.

Children with clefts of the secondary palate may have speech problems similar to cases with total clefts of the primary and secondary palate (*described below*).

Clefts Involving both the Primary and Secondary Palates

These may be unilateral (*Fig.* 20.1*b*) (if primary palate involved on one side only) or bilateral (*Fig.* 20.1*c*) (if primary palate involved on both sides). These cases present the greatest problems: surgical, dental, orthodontic and speech. Superimposed upon the normal range of factors which can give rise to malocclusion are the maxillary deformity, the repaired upper lip and the dental anomalies in the region of the cleft which all contribute to the malocclusion. A detailed account of bilateral complete clefts is not given because the problems are in general similar to those of unilateral cases, but mention is made of differences where appropriate.

SKELETAL RELATIONSHIP

Not only is there tissue deficiency but maxillary growth is adversely affected and skeletal malrelationships often become more severe as the child grows.

Antero-posterior

The anteroposterior deficiency of the maxilla gives rise to a Class III skeletal pattern and often to a Class III incisor relationship.

Vertical

A discrepancy in the vertical plane is often not evident at an early age but becomes increasingly apparent with growth, and the premolars and permanent canines may fail to erupt into occlusion. In unilateral cases the lesser segment is mainly affected, but both sides may be involved in bilateral cases.

The vertical anomaly is associated in part with a general lack of downward and forward growth of the maxilla and in part with a localized failure of alveolar development.

Transverse

In a unilateral cleft the teeth on the lesser segment almost always exhibit some degree of lingual occlusion. There may also be a crossbite on the other side. In bilateral cases both buccal segments are often in crossbite.

SOFT TISSUES

It is difficult to describe the soft tissues in conventional terms. The upper lip tends to cover more of the upper incisors than normal and it is often tight, showing a reduced area of vermilion border. The lip is tight due to lack of tissue and the surgical repair, and this has a bearing on the upper incisor position.

The nose is also affected in most cases of cleft lip. The nostril on the side involved is wide and the ala flattened.

OCCLUSAL FEATURES

The upper arch is often crowded and in unilateral cases there is a shift of centre line to the affected side. In bilateral cases the premaxilla is often markedly malpositioned. Local dental anomalies at the site of the cleft are similar to those found in clefts of the primary palate (*described above*).

Overjet

The upper central incisors are frequently retroclined and in lingual occlusion. This relationship often becomes worse with growth.

Overbite

In the younger child, the overbite may sometimes be deep but it becomes reduced as the face grows. However, in cases where there is an anterior displacement of the mandible and overclosure, the overbite will be deep.

Buccal Segments

The upper arch is often crowded and early loss of deciduous molars will lead to rapid loss of space. Impaction of maxillary first permanent molars is sometimes a contributory factor to the loss of second deciduous molars. There is frequently a Class III buccal segment relationship. A lateral open bite may be found (in unilateral cases on the side of the lesser segment; in bilateral cases on both sides). Unilateral and bilateral crossbites are common. The upper permanent canine on the side of the cleft is frequently palatally positioned and in infra-occlusion.

MANDIBULAR POSITIONS AND PATHS OF CLOSURE

The lack of vertical growth of the maxilla results, in some cases, in an increase in freeway space so that there is a degree of over-closure. If there is a premature contact in the incisor region, a forward displacement of the mandible will also be found. Many cleft palate cases have lateral mandibular displacements associated with a crossbite.

TREATMENT OF CLEFTS INVOLVING BOTH THE PRIMARY AND SECONDARY PALATES

Surgery

The objectives of surgery are to allow the patient to (1) look well, (2) speak well, (3) function adequately.

The Lip

Most clefts are repaired between 6 and 12 weeks of age. The alveolar cleft may also be repaired at this time.

The Palate

Clefts of the hard and soft palate are usually repaired at about 18 months of age. Some surgeons prefer to operate at an earlier age (6–12 months) before the child develops adaptive speech habits. Others repair the soft palate at 18 months but delay the hard palate repair until further maxillary growth has taken place.

Surgical Revision

The child often has to undergo secondary operations to the nose, lip or palate. This must be taken into account in planning the dental management.

Pre-surgical Treatment (Orthopaedics)

In the infant with a unilateral cleft of lip and palate the greater and lesser segments may be malrelated: they may be widely separated or over-lapping or somewhere in between. In bilateral cases the pre-maxilla is often far forwards of the lateral segments.

Some surgeons consider that the surgical repair of the lip is easier to do if the segments are aligned before surgery. Presurgical orthopaedic treatment may be undertaken in order to improve the alignment of the segments. Whether such treatment produces better long term results is a matter of controversy.

Presurgical orthopaedic treatment is performed by fitting either a hard ar a soft acrylic plate. The hard acrylic plate is designed to mould the gum pads into position and is usually supported by a headcap. In bilateral cases, the headcap may be used to apply distal traction to the protruding premaxilla. (*Fig.* 20.2). Soft acrylic plates are trimmed (eased) on the palatal surfaces to allow the segments to align as growth takes place (Hotz et al., 1978).

Dental Management

This will be discussed under the headings of routine dental care; orthodontic treatment; restorative treatment—bridgework or partial dentures.

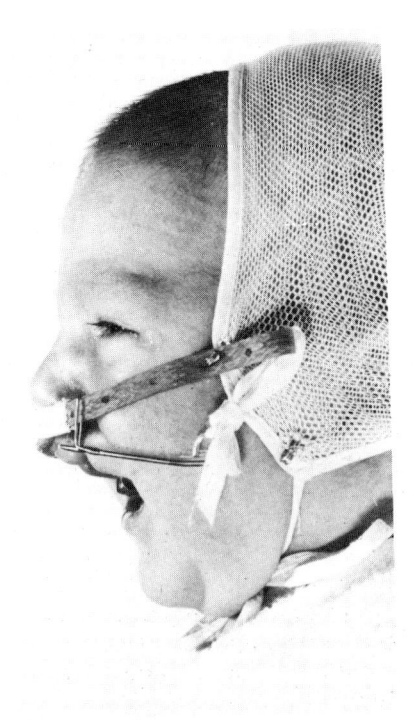

Fig. 20.2. Bilateral cleft lip and palate patient showing strapping attached to headcap to reposition premaxilla. It is important for the patient to wear intra-oral appliance to prevent collapse of the lateral segments.

Routine Dental Care

Before the child is operated on general discussion should be held with the parents about diet, oral hygiene and the importance of regular dental inspections. The possibility of orthodontic treatment at a later stage should be explained. Preventive measures should be arranged, e.g. the prescription of fluoride tablets from birth (in low fluoride areas) and the later application of topical fluoride and fissure sealants.

Children with cleft palates have particular problems in maintaining good oral hygiene. The natural cleansing action of lips, cheeks and tongue appears to be less effective and the presence of crowded and rotated teeth and the lack of good occlusion add to the patient's problems. Thus the importance of effective oral hygiene measures must be emphasized from the outset.

Orthodontic Treatment

The objectives of treatment are the same as those of surgery: viz. that appearance, speech and function should be as good as the circumstances allow. No orthodontic treatment is advised until the permanent incisors erupt. The child should be seen at regular intervals for routine dental checks and treatment.

Treatment in the early mixed dentition. Only treatment which will be stable should be carried out at this stage. The operator should also ensure that the treatment proposed will not merely add to the general problems of the child or parent.

1. Correction of lingually placed permanent incisors should be undertaken provided that there is an overbite which will retain the tooth movement.

2. Supernumerary or malposed teeth may have to be removed surgically.

Lateral expansion of the upper arch should *not* be undertaken at this stage as it will not be stable.

Treatment in the early permanent dentition. A full diagnosis and treatment plan must be formulated. The child's general dental condition, cooperation, travelling difficulties, and the limits set by the skeletal pattern and soft tissues must be taken into consideration.

Treatment varies according to the severity of the case.

1. Where there are reasonable arches with minimal antero-posterior discrepancies and a sound dentition, orthodontic treatment, ideally followed by bridgework to replace missing or malformed teeth, is indicated.

2. Where the discrepancy in arch relationship is moderate or the patient is not suitable for complex appliance treatment, it is often best to remove poorly formed and malpositioned teeth and to fit a metal denture to give a reasonable appearance without damaging the soft tissues.

3. In severe cases where orthodontic and prosthetic techniques alone will not give a satisfactory aesthetic result, surgery to improve the patient's profile may be indicated. This will usually involve the maxilla and sometimes a combined maxillary/mandibular operation. Surgery may be preceded or followed by orthodontic treatment and finally restorative procedures.

Rapid expansion in cleft palate cases. Rapid expansion of the upper arch is sometimes indicated in order to improve the arch form and buccal segment relationship with the lower teeth. The expansion is rapid so that the maxillary segments, rather than the teeth, are moved. However, it can be difficult to control precisely the direction of the expansion force; and although the expansion is rapidly achieved, it will not be stable unless it is permanently retained. Rapid expansion is undertaken using cast cap splints cemented to the teeth and a large Fischer screw activated two or three times each day.

Restorative Treatment

The long term restorative plan should be considered before orthodontic treatment is begun. It may be possible to simplify orthodontic treatment, if for example a rotated tooth is to be incorporated as an abutment in a bridge.

An acrylic partial denture is not a satisfactory long term prosthesis for the cleft palate patient: it merely adds to the difficulties in maintaining a good standard of oral hygiene and a healthy palatal mucosa. On the other hand, bridgework is not indicated for the patient with poor oral hygiene and a poor standard of dental care. Before advanced restorative treatment is undertaken it is important that the patient should be willing and able to maintain a good standard of oral hygiene. The importance of adequate dental care must be emphasized from the earliest possible stage.

Speech. Cleft palate patients have speech problems, in part because the soft palate tends to be rather short and lacking in mobility, so that during speech there is a nasal escape of air. Many also have hearing defects due to middle ear infections. Speech therapy is an important part of the total treatment. Despite their difficulties, a remarkably high proportion of these children have quite good speech.

CONCLUSION

The surgical, orthodontic and speech problems of cleft palate children are treated by a team of specialists. The general dental practitioner should also be part of that team. He must concentrate on preventive dental measures and early treatment of carious lesions. Only if the child is dentally motivated and enjoys a high standard of dental care can the best be done for him by the other members of the team.

References

Hotz M. M., Gnoinski W. M., Nussbaumer H. et al. (1978) Early maxillary orthopedics in CLP cases: guidelines for surgery. *Cleft Palate Journal* **15**, 405–411.

Ross R. B. and Johnston M. C. (1972) *Cleft Lip and Palate.* Baltimore, Williams & Wilkins.

Appendix I

Orthodontic Diagnosis and Treatment Planning

1. Introduction and History

Age and sex.
Reason for attendance.
Previous illnesses and accidents.
Habits.
Assessment of interest and co-operation.

2. Soft Tissue Morphology and Muscle Behaviour Patterns

Lips

a. Morphology.
  i. Competent or incompetent.
  ii. Habitual position. Whether together or apart.
  iii. Lip lines: upper, lower and active.
b. Behaviour. The amount of circumoral contraction during speech, expressive behaviour and swallowing.

Tongue

a. Size.
b. Position, e.g. tongue resting forwards between the incisors against the lower lip.
c. Swallowing behaviour: typical or atypical.

3. Skeletal Relationships

Assessed clinically and verified from lateral skull radiographs if available.

4. Mandibular Position and Path of Closure

  a. Mandibular position: rest or habit posture.
  b. Interocclusal clearance or freeway space.
  c. Path of closure: hinge movement from rest, or deviation or displacement.

5. Intra-oral Examination

Clinical examination aided by models and radiographs.

a. *General Condition of Mouth*

Teeth present:
  i. Erupted and unerupted.
  ii. Missing teeth (extracted/developmentally missing).
  iii. Extra teeth (supernumerary/supplemental).
  iv. Ectopic teeth and pathological conditions (odontomes, cysts etc.).

Oral hygiene. Good, average, poor.
Peridontal condition.
Condition of teeth:
  i. Caries rate.
  ii. Damaged teeth/malformed teeth.
  iii. Non-vital teeth discoloration; periapical involvement.
  iv. Resorption.

b. *Tooth Positions and Relationships*

Upper and lower labial segments:
  i. Inclinations and rotations.
  ii. Crowding/spacing.
  iii. Relationship—midline; overbite; overjet.

Upper and lower buccal segments:
  i. Inclinations and rotations.
  ii. Crowding/spacing.
  iii. Relationship—antero-posterior, lateral, vertical.

6. Diagnosis

Summary of salient features elicited in the case assessment (*see* 1–3 inclusive above).

Treatment plan. This is decided from the diagnosis, a stable final position for the teeth being all important. The co-operation of the patient and parents must also be taken into consideration.

Treatment may be: (*a*) ideal; (*b*) palliative.

Practical:
- *a*. General treatment: conservative, periodontal, etc.
- *b*. Orthodontic treatment: timing and expected duration, extractions, appliances, retention, prognosis.

Appendix II

Definitions

1. Soft Tissues

Competent Lips	A lip seal is maintained with minimal muscular effort when the mandible is in the rest position.
Incompetent Lips	With the mandible in the rest position muscular effort is required to obtain a lip seal.
Anterior Oral Seal	A seal produced by contact between the lips or between the tongue and lower lip.
Posterior Oral Seal	A seal between the soft palate and dorsum of the tongue.

2. Teeth and Occlusion

Ideal Occlusion	A theoretical occlusion based on the morphology of the teeth.
Normal Occlusion	An occlusion which satisfies the requirements of function and aesthetics but in which there are minor irregularities of individual teeth.
Malocclusion	An occlusion in which there is a malrelationship between the arches in any of the planes of space or in which there are anomalies in tooth position beyond the limits of normal.
Centric Occlusion	A position of maximal intercuspation which is a position of centric relation.
Overjet	The relationship between upper and lower incisors in the horizontal plane.

DEFINITIONS

Overbite	The overlap of the lower incisors by the upper incisors in the vertical plane.
Complete Overbite	An overbite in which the lower incisors contact either the upper incisors or the palatal mucosa.
Incomplete Overbite	An overbite in which the lower incisors contact neither the upper incisors nor the palatal mucosa.
Anterior Open Bite	The lower incisors are not overlapped in the vertical plane by the upper incisors and do not occlude with them.
Labial Segments	The incisor teeth.
Buccal Segments	The canine, premolar and molar teeth.
Cingulum Plateau	The middle part of the palatal surface of the upper incisor.
Incisor Classification	A classification based on the incisor relationship in the antero-posterior axis (*see* pp. 52–53).
Angle's Classification	A classification of malocclusion based on arch relationship in the antero-posterior axis (*see* pp. 48–50).
Crossbite	A transverse discrepancy in arch relationship. The lower arch is wider than the upper so that the buccal cusps of the lower teeth occlude outside the buccal cusps of the corresponding upper teeth. May also be used for total lingual occlusion of the lower buccal teeth.
Scissors Bite	A lingual crossbite of the lower teeth.
Leeway Space	The excess space provided when the deciduous canine and molars are replaced by the permanent canine and premolars. The leeway space is slightly greater in the lower arch.

Primate Spacing	A naturally occurring spacing in the deciduous dentition, mesial to the upper canine and distal to the lower canine.
Diastema	A natural spacing between teeth.
Dens in Dente	An enamel-lined invagination sometimes present on the palatal surface of the upper incisors.
Dilaceration	The deformed development of a tooth as a result of disturbance of the relationship between the uncalcified and already calcified portions of a developing tooth.

3. Skeletal Relationships, Mandibular Positions and Paths of Closure

Alveolar Process	The parts of the maxilla and mandible the development and presence of which depend on the presence of the teeth.
Skeletal Bases	The maxilla and mandible excluding the alveolar processes.
Skeletal Pattern	The relationship between the mandible and maxilla in the antero-posterior axis.
Intermaxillary Space	The space between the upper and lower skeletal bases when the mandible is in the rest position.
Bimaxillary	Pertaining to both upper and lower jaws.
Prognathism	The projection of the jaws from beneath the cranial base.
Positions of Centric Relation	The relationships between the mandible and maxilla when the condyles are in retruded unstrained positions in the glenoid fossae.
Rest Position	The position of the mandible in which the muscles acting on it

DEFINITIONS

	show minimal activity. Essentially it is determined by the resting lengths of the muscles of mastication and it is a position of centric relation.
Habit Posture	A postured position of the mandible habitually maintained either to facilitate the production of an anterior oral seal or for aesthetic reasons.
Interocclusal Clearance	The space between the occlusal surfaces of the teeth when the mandible is in the rest position or a position of habitual posture.
Freeway Space	The interocclusal clearance when the mandible is in the rest position.
Deviation of the Mandible	A sagittal movement of the mandible during closure from a habit posture to a position of centric occlusion.
Displacement of the Mandible	A sagittal or lateral displacement of the mandible as a result of a premature contact.
Premature Contact	An occlusal contact which occurs during the centric path of closure of the mandible before maximal cuspal occlusion is reached. This may result in either displacement of the mandible or movement of the tooth or both.

4. Cephalometric Points and Planes

Anterior Nasal Spine (ANS)	The tip of the anterior nasal spine.
Articulare (Ar)	The projection on a lateral skull radiograph of the posterior outline of the condylar process onto the inferior outline of the cranial base.

Glabella	The most prominent point over the frontal bone.
Gnathion (Gn)	The most anterior inferior point on the bony chin.
Gonion (Go)	The most posterior inferior point at the angle of the mandible.
Menton (Me)	The most inferior point on the bony chin.
Nasion (N)	The most anterior point on the frontonasal suture.
Orbitale (Or)	The lowest point on the bony margin of the orbit.
Pogonion (Pog)	The most anterior point on the bony chin.
Point A	The deepest point on the maxillary profile between Anterior Nasal Spine and the alveolar crest.
Point B	The deepest point on the mandibular profile between the pogonion and the alveolar crest.
Porion (Po)	The uppermost outermost point on the bony external acoustic meatus.
Posterior Nasal Spine (PNS)	The tip of the posterior nasal spine.
Sella (S)	The mid-point of the sella turcica.
Frankfort Plane	The plane through the orbitale and porion. This is meant to approximate the horizontal plane when the head is in the free postural position but this varies appreciably.
Mandibular Plane	The plane through menton and tangent to the inferior border of the angle of the mandible (or alternatively through the gonion).
Maxillary Plane	The plane through ANS and PNS.

Index

Adams' clasp, 65–7
Aesthetic line, 26
Alveolar bone, normal, 54
   process, 206
Anchorage, 67–9
Andresen appliance, 173–5
Angle's classification of
       malocclusion, 48–53,
       205
Anodontia, 94
Anterior bite planes, 70–1
  nasal spine (ANS), 17, 208
  open bite, 131–2, 205
    in class III malocclusion,
      (*Fig.* 12.1) 129, 154, 161
    surgery for, 184
    swallowing behaviour and,
      31
  oral seal, 204
Appliances,
  fixed *see* Fixed appliances
  functional, *see* Functional
    appliances
  influence on maxillary growth,
    8
  removable, *see* Removable
    appliances
Archwires for fixed appliances,
    164, (*Fig.* 17.3) 166
Articulare, 208
Attachments for fixed
    appliances,163, (*Figs.*
    17.1–2) 164–5
Auxiliaries for fixed appliances,
    164

Bands for fixed appliances, 163,
    (*Fig.* 17.3) 166
Baseplate, 69–71
  repairing, 73
Begg appliance, (*Fig.* 17.3) 166,
    169
Bite planes, 70–1
Bone, changes from pressure,
    56–7
  see also Alveolar bone
Bows, labial, 64, 65
Buccal segment, 205
  distal movement, 143–4
  malrelationships, 128
    class II division 1, 142
    class II division 2, 148
    class III, 155
    transverse, 132–4
    vertical, 129
  retraction, 81–2, 119, 143–4
Buccal spring, 64
  for canine retraction, (*Fig.*
    9.3a) 78

Canines, buccal movement of, 87
  deciduous, early loss of, 97
    extraction of, 126
    retained, 109
  extraction to relieve crowding,
    125
  lower, crowding of, 120–1
    retraction of, 89–90
  palatal movement of, 86–7

Canines (*cont.*)
  upper, crowded, 124–5
    extraction of, 178–9
    retraction of, 75–9, 144
    surgery for, 177–9
    transplantation of, 179
    see also Buccal segment
Cantilever spring, (*Fig.* 8.1) 62
Centric relation, 34, 207
Cephalometric radiograph,
      analysis, 17–26
  interpretation, 24–5
  landmarks, 17–21
  measurement from, 24
  obtaining, (*Fig.* 2.5) 16, 17
  reference lines and planes,
      (*Fig.* 2.7) 19, 21–3,
      208–9
Cingulum plateau, 205
Clasps, 65–7
  modified, 169, (*Fig.* 17.5) 170
  repairing, 73
Cleft lip and palate, 190–1
  aetiology, 190
  classification, 190–1
  mandibular positions and
      paths of closure, 195
  occlusal features, 194–5
  skeletal relationships, 193
  soft tissues in, 193–4
  supernumerary teeth in, 111
  treatment, 195–200
Cleft palate, causing unilateral
      crossbite, 134
Cranial base, 5–8
  vault, 5
Crossbite, 205
  bilateral, 132–3
    in class III malocclusion,
      (*Fig.* 12.1) 129, 132–3,
      155, 161
  correction by posterior bite
      plane, 71
  unilateral, 133–4
    in class III malocclusion,
      155, 161

Crowding, 118–27
  canine, 120–1, 124–5
  causing early loss of deciduous
      teeth, 98
  incisor, 120–1, 124–5
    causes of, 13, 14
    increase in, 44
  lower arch, 120–4, 137, 143
  molars, 122–4, 125–6
  reduction by attrition, 46
  upper arch, 124–6, 137, 143,
      151–2, 154, 160

Deciduous dentition,
      development, 37–9
  early loss, 97–9
  extraction to relieve crowding,
      126–7
  orthodontic treatment timing,
      2
  retained, 108–13
Dens-in-dente, 113, 206
Dental arch, at birth 36
  changes in relationships in
      permanent occlusion, 45
  growth, 38–9
  increasing, 118
  malrelationships, 12–14, 47,
      128–34
  relationship, 14–16
  see also Mandibular arch;
      Maxillary arch
Dental groove, 36
Dento-alveolar adaptation, 13–14
  compensation, 12–13
  surgery, 182–4
Dento-skeletal relationships, 25
Depression of teeth, 55
Diastema, 206
  median, from persistent
      fraenum, 115–16
    from supernumerary teeth,
      112
    with incisor eruption, 41

Dilaceration, 114, 206
Displacement of individual teeth, 47, 114
Disto-occlusion, 49
Drifting, molar, 50

Ectodermal dysplasia, 94, 95
Edgewise appliance, (*Fig.* 17.2) 165, 168
Elastics, 64, (*Fig.* 8.3) 65, 164
En Masse appliance, 68
  for retraction of upper buccal segments, 81–2
Extraction
  to balance loss of
    deciduous canines, 97, 99
    deciduous molars, 98, 99
  of first permanent molars, 102–8
  to relieve crowding, 96, 106–7, 119
    in lower arch, 120–4, 137, 143, 160
    in upper arch, 124–6, 137, 143, 151–2, 160
  serial, 126–7
  of upper canines, 178–9
Extra-oral anchorage, 68–9
  for canine retraction, 77, (*Fig.* 9.3) 78
  in class II division 1 treatment, 144

Face, growth of, 5–14
  height assessment, 16
Facebow, 68, (*Fig.* 8.5) 69, 169
Facial line, 21
Fixed appliances, 163–71
  advantages and disadvantages, 167
  causing bodily movement of teeth, 54
  components, 163–6

Fixed appliances (*cont.*)
  limitations, 167–8
  techniques, 168–9
  with removable appliances, 169–70
Fraenectomy, 181
Fraenum, upper labial, 116–17
Fränkel appliance, 175–6
Frankfort plane, angle
  assessment, 16
  in class III malocclusion, 157
  definition, 21, 208
Freeway space, 34, 207
Functional appliances, 172–6
  influence on mandibular growth, 9

Gemination, 113
Gingiva, recession in class III malocclusion, 159
  traumatized in class II division 2 malocclusion, 150
Gingival groove, 36
Gingivitis, hyperplastic, 142
  mouth-breathing, 142
Glabella, 208
Gnathion (Gn), 19, 208
Gonion (Go), 17–19, 208
Gum pads at birth, 36

Habits, causing malocclusion, 114–16, 134, 142
  posture, 207
Headcap, 68, (*Fig.* 8.5) 69
  for cleft lip and palate, (*Fig.* 20.2) 197
Headgear, 68–9, 93
Hyperplasia, gingival, 142
  unilateral condylar, 134
Hypodontia, 95–6

Impaction, 177, 179
Incision inferius (II), 19
  superius (IS), 19
Incisors, alignment of labial bow, 77
  classification, 52–3, 205
  deciduous, early loss of, 97
    retained, 108–9
  development, deciduous, 36–8
    permanent, 39–41
  extrusion, 161
  inclination assessment, 25, 28–9
  lower, crowded, 13, 14, 44, 120–1
    extraction, 120–1
    proclination, 153
    proclined, 14
    retroclination, 14
  overbite *see* Overbite
  overjet *see* Overjet
  retraction by anterior bite plane, 70, (*Fig.* 8.6) 71
  unerupted, 181
  upper, approximation of central, 75
    correction of instanding, 71
    crowded, 124–5
    dilaceration, 114
    extraction, 125
    fractured, 142
    lateral alignment, 152–3
    lateral used as central, 102
    loss of, 100–2
    mesiodens causing problems with, 112
    missing lateral, 95–6
    proclination, 84–6, 153
    proclined, 12–13, 28, 161
    retraction, 82–4, 143–6
    retroclination, 12–13
  see also Labial segment
Inclination of individual teeth, 47
Infradentals (Id), 20
Infra-occlusion, 47
Intermaxillary anchorage, 68

Intermaxillary (*cont.*)
  space, 206
    assessment of, 15–16
    growth of, (*Fig.* 2.2) 7, 13
Interocclusal clearance, 207
Intramaxillary anchorage, 68
Intra-oral examination, 202

J hooks, 68, (*Fig.* 9.3*b*) 78
Jaw, malrelationship, adaptation to, 13–14
  compensation for, 12
  relationship, assessment of, 14–16
    skeletal growth influences on, 7–8

Köle procedure, 184

Labial bows, 64, 65, 83–4
  fraenum, upper, 116–17
  for incisor retraction, 77–9
  segments, 205
    in class I malocclusion, 135
    in class II division 1 malocclusion, 158
    in class II division 2 malocclusion, 147–8
    in class III malocclusion, 154
  malrelationships, 128
  surgery for, 182–4
  vertical, 130–2
  set-back mandibular ostectomy, lower, 183
  set-down, lower, 184
  set-up, lower, 184
Lateral open bite, 129
  skull radiograph *see* Cephalometric radiograph
  sulcus, 36

Leeway space, 42, 306
Lip, cleft *see* Cleft lip
  morphology, at birth, 36
    in class II division 2
      malocclusion, 150
    competent, 27, 204
    effect on malocclusion, 12,
      15
    incompetent, (*Fig.* 3.1*b*) 26,
      27, 204
      causing overjet relapse,
        146
      in class II division 1
        malocclusion, (*Fig.* 14.2)
        140, 141
      in class III malocclusion,
        158
      swallowing behaviour and,
        30, 141, 158

Malocclusion, 46–53, 204
  aetiology, 53
    local factors in, 94–117
  class I, (*Fig.* 2.4*a*) 12, 48,
    135–7
    extraction of first permanent
      molars in, 106–7
    labial segments, 135
    occlusal features, 135
    skeletal relationships, 135–6
    soft tissues in, 136
    treatment, 137
  class II, (*Fig.* 2.4*b*) 12, 15, 49
    cephalometric analysis,
      (*Fig.* 2.8) 22
    division 1, 49, 130, 138–46
      Andresen appliance for,
        173–5
      Fränkel appliance for, 176
      labial segments in, 138
      mandibular positions and
        paths of closure, 34, 141
      occlusal features, 138

Malocclusion, division 1, (*cont.*)
    skeletal relationships,
      139–41
    soft tissues in, 141
    treatment, 142–6
  division 2, 49, (*Fig.* 6.3) 50,
    130, 147–53
    conversion from division
      1, 145
    mandibular positions and
      paths of closure, 35, 149
    occlusal features, 147–8
    skeletal relationships,
      148–9
    soft tissues in, 150
    treatment, 150–3
  extraction of first permanent
    molars in, 107–8
class III, (*Fig.* 2.4*c*) 12, 15, 50
  (*Fig.* 6.4) 51, 154–62
  anterior open bite in,
    (*Fig.* 12.1) 129, 131
  crossbite in, (*Fig.* 12.1) 129,
    132–3
  extraction of first permanent
    molars in, 108
  mandibular position and
    paths of closure in, 35,
    158
  occlusal features, 154–5
  skeletal relationships, 155–8
  soft tissue in, 158
  surgery for, 183
  treatment, 159–62
classification, 48–53
definition, 1
due to anomalies in form and
  position of teeth, 113–4
due to anomalies in number of
  teeth, 94–113
due to habits, 114–16
transverse, 132–4
vertical, 129–32
Mandible, deviations of, 35, 207
  displacements of, 35, 115, 134,
    207

Mandible (*cont.*)
  growth of, (*Fig.* 2.2) 7, 8–11
  growth rotations of, (*Fig.* 2.3) 10, 13–14
  positions and paths of closure of, 34–5
    assessment, 202
    definition, 206–7
Mandibular arch, crowded, 120–4, 137
  treatment in class I malocclusion, 137
  in class II division 1 malocclusion, 143
  in class II division 2 malocclusion, 151
  in class III malocclusion, 159–60
  ostectomy, lower labial setback, 183
  osteotomy, 186–7
  plane, angle assessment, 16
    definition, 21, 208
  prognathism, 186–7
  retrognathism, 187–8
  retrusion, 12–13
Maxilla, growth of, (*Fig.* 2.2) 7, 8
Maxillary arch, crowded, 124–6, 137
  expansion, 88–9, 199
  narrowing due to thumb sucking, 115
  treatment in class I malocclusion, 137
  in class II division 1 malocclusion, 143–6
  in class II division 2 malocclusion, 151–2
  in class III malocclusion, 160–2
  ostectomy, anterior, 184
  plane, definition, 21–2, 208
Menton (Me), 20, 208
Mesial drift, causing crowding, 44
Mesiodens, 110, 111–12

Mills' bow, (*Fig.* 9.9) 84
Mixed dentition, development of, 39–43
  early, orthodontic treatment of, 3, 198
  extraction of first permanent molar in, 103–5, 106
  late, orthodontic treatment timing of, 3
Molars, crowded, (*Fig.* 11.1) 119
  deciduous, early loss of, 97–8
    extraction of, 127
    retained, 109
    submerged, 96, 109–10
  development, deciduous, (*Table* 5.1) 38
    permanent, (*Table* 5.2) 40, 42–3
  distal movement of first permanent, 80–1
  drifting, 50
  extraction to relieve crowding, 123–4, 125–6
  first permanent, loss of, 102–8
  lower, crowded, 122–4
    distal movement of first, 90–1
    surgery on third, 179–80
  missing third, 95
  upper, crowded, 126
  see also Buccal segment
Multiband techniques, 168

Nasion (N), 208
Neckstrap, 68
Neutro-occlusion, 48

Obwegeser technique, 186–7
Occlusal plane, definition of, 22
Occlusion, centric, 205
  changes occurring in permanent, 44–5

Occlusion (*cont.*)
  definition of, 204–6
  facial growth effects on, 11
  ideal, 1, 204
  normal, 1, 204
    development, 36–45
Open bite *see under* Anterior *and* Lateral
Oral health, 142
  screen, 172–3
  seal, 204
  surgery, dento-alveolar, 182–4
    for cleft lip and palate, 195–6, 199
    major, 184–8
    minor, 177–81
Orbitale (Or), 20, 208
Orthodontics (general),
    cephalometric analysis and, 23
  definition of, 1
  diagnosis and treatment planning, Appendix 1, 201–3
  for cleft lip and palate, 198–200
  scope and aims of, 1
  timing of treatment, 2–4, 14
Ostectomy, anterior maxillary, 184
  lower labial set-back mandibular, 183
Osteotomy, vertical subsigmoid, 186–7
Overbite, 205
  in cleft lip and palate, 194
  complete, 205
    in class II division 2 malocclusion, 147–8
  incomplete, 205
  in class II division 1 malocclusion, 138, (*Fig.* 14.2) 140
    from endogenous tongue thrust, 32
    from thumb sucking, 115, 138

Overbite, in class II (*cont.*)
    from swallowing behaviour, 31, 138
  increased, occlusal factors in, 130
    skeletal factors in, 130
    surgery for, 184
  reduced, in class III malocclusion, 154, 161
  reduction by anterior bite plane, 70, 130–2
    in class II division 1 malocclusion, 144
    in class II division 2 malocclusion, 150, 152
Overclosure, from sagittal displacement of mandible, 35
Overeruption of buccal segments, 129
Overjet, 205
  in cleft lip and palate, 194
  increased, (*Fig.* 14.1) 139
    in class II division 2 malocclusion, 147
    from endogenous tongue thrust, 31–2
    from thumb sucking, 115
    reduction in class II division 1 malocclusion, 145
    with oral screen, 172
    swallowing behaviour and, 31
  reduced in class III malocclusion, 160
  reverse, 154, 160–1
  small, reduction by labial bow, 77, (*Fig.* 9.4) 79
  stability of correction, 146, 162

Pain, in class II division 2 malocclusion, 149
  in class III malocclusion, 159
Palatal spring, (*Fig.* 8.2) 63

Palatal spring (*cont.*)
  for canine retraction, (*Fig.* 9.2) 76
Palate, cleft *see* Cleft palate
Patient cooperation, 167, 200
Peg-shaped tooth, 113
Pericision, (*Fig.* 7.2) 57
Pericoronitis, 123
Periodontium, tension and compression within, caused by tooth movement within, 55–8
Permanent dentition, development of, 43–5
  early, orthodontic treatment timing of, 3
  late, orthodontic treatment timing of, 4
Pierre Robin syndrome, 192
Plate, for cleft lip and palate, 196
Pogonion (Pog), 20, 208
Point A, 20, 208
  B, 20–1, 208
Porion (Po), 21, 208
Posterior bite planes, 71
  nasal spine (PNS), 20, 208
  oral seal, 204
Premature contact, 207
Premolars, buccal movement of, 87
  development of, (*Table* 5.2) 40, 42
  drifting following loss of first permanent molar, 103, (*Fig.* 10.5) 104
  extraction to relieve crowding, 120, 122, 124, 126, 127
  lower, crowded, 121–2
  missing second, 96
  palatal movement of, 86–7
  retraction, 79–80
  upper, crowded, 125–6
  see also Buccal segment
Primate spacings, 38, 206
Proclination, bimaxillary, 29
  of lower incisors, causes of, 14

Proclination (*cont.*)
  of upper incisors, causes of, 12, 28
  results of, 13
Prognathism, 9, 186–7, 207
Prosthion (Pr), 21
Pulp death, 59

Removable appliances, acrylic resin, 73
  adjustment of, 93
  advantages and disadvantages, 167
  anchorage, 67–9
  baseplate, 69–71
  causing tipping, 54
  components, 61–73
  construction and repair, 72–3
  design, 74, (*Fig.* 9.1) 75
  instructions to patients for, 92–3
  lower, 89–91
  passive, 91–2
  principles of, 61
  retention, 65–7
  upper, for labial or palatal tooth movements, 82–9
    for mesial or distal tooth movements, 75–82
  with fixed appliances, 169–70
Retainers, 92, 172
Retention, 65–7
Retractor, Roberts', 64
Retroclination, bimaxillary, 29
  of lower incisors, results of, 13, 14
  of upper incisors, from mandibular retrusion, 12
Retrognathism, 187–8
Roberts' retractor, 82–3
Root, ankylosis, 109–10, 179
  bent, 114
  filling, 179

Root (*cont.*)
  resorption, 59
Rotation of individual teeth, 47

Sagittal splitting technique, 186–7
Scissors bite, 205
Screw plate, 85–6
Screws, 64
Sella (S), 208
Skeletal bases, 206
  growth of face and skull, 5–14
  patterns, (*Fig.* 2.4) 12, 206
    assessment of, 15
    relationships, 14–16, 201, 206–7
Skull,
  growth of, 5–14
  radiograph, lateral *see* Cephalometric radiograph
Soft tissues, definition of, 204
  morphology, 27–33
    assessment of, 15, 25–6, 201
    effects on malocclusion, 12, 134
    in class I malocclusion, 136
    in class II division 1 malocclusion, 141
    in class II division 2 malocclusion, 150
    in class III malocclusion, 158
  surgery planning and, 185
Southend clasp, (*Fig.* 8.4*b*) 66, 67
Space maintainers, 91
  for early loss of deciduous teeth, 99, (*Fig.* 10.2) 100
  for loss of upper incisor, (*Fig.* 10.3) 101
Spacing, 118
Speech problems, 200

Springs, 61–4
  repair, 73
Stacking, (*Fig.* 11.1) 119, 126
Supernumerary teeth, 110–11, 180–1
Supplemental teeth, 111
Supra-occlusion, 47
Swallowing behaviour, adaptive atypical, 30–1
  adult, 29
  infantile, 29
  persistent, 30
  primary atypical, 31–2, 141

T springs, 84–5, (*Fig.* 9.14) 88
Thumb sucking causing malocclusion, 114–16, 134, 142
Tilting of individual teeth, 47
Tipping, 54, (*Fig.* 7.1) 55, 56, 67
Tissue changes with tooth movement, 54–60
Tongue, endogenous thrust, 31–2
  morphology, 29–30
  swallowing behaviour, 29–32
Tooth (general), anomalies of form and position in, 113–14
  developmentally missing, 94–6
  loss of permanent, 99–108
  malpositioned, 47, 114
  movement, areas of pressure from, 56
    areas of tension from, 56–8
    harmful effects of, 59
    rate of, 58–9
    resistance to, 67
    tissue changes from, 55
    types of, 54–5
  supernumerary, 110, 111–2, 180–1
Tooth-arch disproportion, 118–27

Trepanation, lateral, 179–80

Ugly duckling dentition, 41,
    (*Fig.* 5.3) 42

Wassmund procedure, 184
Whip, 170, (*Fig.* 17.6) 171
Wire stops, 70